## Practice Questions

1. A 45-year-old male comes to the emergency room after being involved in a head-on motor vehicle accident earlier in the day. The patient notes that he struck his head, but he did not experience any loss of consciousness. His blood pressure is 190/110, his respirations are irregular, and his electrocardiogram (EKG) shows sinus bradycardia with a heart rate of 42 beats per minute. The patient's symptoms are part of which clinical triad?
    a. Beck's triad
    b. Charcot's triad
    c. Cushing's triad
    d. Bergman's triad

2. All of the following are minor manifestations of acute rheumatic fever as described by the modified Jones criteria EXCEPT
    a. Erythema marginatum
    b. Leukocytosis
    c. Elevated erythrocyte sedimentation rate (ESR)
    d. thralgia

3. A 19-year-old woman comes to the office complaining of a painful rash on her elbows and knees. The rash appears as raised erythematous areas topped with silvery, scaling skin. She reports, "The rash is very itchy." She had similar symptoms several weeks before, but they spontaneously resolved without treatment. Which of the following is most likely to be the diagnosis?
    a. Impetigo
    b. Tinea corporis
    c. Rosacea
    d. Psoriasis

4. During a colonoscopy, the gastroenterologist notices that the patient's colon wall has a "cobblestone" appearance. Which of the following is the most likely diagnosis?
    a. Celiac sprue
    b. Crohn's disease
    c. Ulcerative colitis
    d. Whipple's disease

5. You are evaluating an obese 37-year-old female in the ER. She has been complaining of right-sided abdominal pain and excessive flatulence. She normally has the pain after eating, but it usually resolves on its own. This episode has persisted for several hours. On physical examination, you palpate her right-upper quadrant while she takes a deep inspiration. Discomfort during this maneuver is referred to as a positive:
    a. Brudziński's sign
    b. Psoas sign
    c. Murphy's sign
    d. Levine's sign

6. You are acting as the first assist in the operating room, and the surgeon asks you to close an abdominal incision with an absorbable suture material. Based on the following choices, which suture would be your pick?
    a. Dermabond
    b. Vicryl
    c. Silk
    d. Nylon

7. All of the following are symptoms of esophageal achalasia EXCEPT
    a. Acid reflux
    b. Dysphagia
    c. Hematochezia
    d. Chest pain

8. Which of the following is NOT part of CREST syndrome?
    a. Calcinosis
    b. Sclerodactyly
    c. Solar urticaria
    d. Esophageal dysmotility

9. A 20-year-old female recently diagnosed with chlamydia comes to your office for swelling and pain in her knees bilaterally. The most likely diagnosis for this woman's complaints is
    a. Sjögren's syndrome
    b. Reiter's syndrome
    c. Turner syndrome
    d. Down syndrome

10. A 26-year-old female comes to the ER with complaints of white vaginal discharge and pelvic pain. She admits to having unprotected sex. On physical examination, she has an inflamed cervix and cervical motion tenderness. Which one of the following two-medication pairs should she receive prior to leaving the ER?
    a. Ceftriaxone 250 mg IM and clindamycin 300 mg po
    b. Clindamycin 300 mg po and azithromycin 1 gm po
    c. Mefoxitin 2 gm IV and azithromycin 1 gm po
    d. Ceftriaxone 250 mg IM and azithromycin 1 gm po

11. A 19-year-old male patient is brought to the ER by his mother for altered mental status. She notes that he "hasn't been acting normally" since the morning. He has a known history of depression and anxiety for which he does not take medication and chronic back pain for which he takes codeine. On physical examination, his pupils are 2 mm bilaterally and he is lethargic, but he is able to be aroused. His heart rate is 44, his blood pressure is 78/44, and his respiratory rate is eight breaths per minute. Which of the following medications may reverse his symptoms and confirm your suspected diagnosis?
    a. Oxycodone
    b. Naloxone
    c. Prednisolone
    d. Buspirone

12. You diagnose an adult patient in your clinic with streptococcal pharyngitis. The patient has a known anaphylactic reaction to penicillin. Which of the following medications would be an acceptable substitute?
   a. Cefepime
   b. Cephalexin
   c. Augmentin
   d. Clarithromycin

13. You are examining a five-year-old patient for a wellness examination. During the examination, you notice that the child has painful-looking, swollen joints and notching of the maxillary incisors. The child has a past medical history of being blind and deaf. Based on his past medical history and examination findings, the patient most likely has a history of
   a. Congenital syphilis
   b. Down syndrome
   c. Osgood–Schlatter disease
   d. Turner syndrome

14. A 45-year-old male presents to your clinic with a painful, erythematous bump on his right eyelid of three days' duration. The eyeball itself is unaffected. His vision is unaffected. He has no crusting on the eyelids or lashes. The most likely diagnosis is
   a. Xanthelasma
   b. Hordeolum
   c. Mongolian spots
   d. Felon

15. A 66-year-old male comes into the office complaining of painless, yellowish, raised patches on his eyelids bilaterally for the past several weeks. He has no other skin lesions and has had no history of these lesions before. He has a known history of hyperlipidemia for which he is noncompliant with medications. What is the most likely diagnosis?
   a. Dermoid cyst
   b. Impetigo
   c. Mongolian spots
   d. Xanthelasma

16. Parents of a five-year-old boy bring him to the ER, noting that he has had worsening ataxia, nausea, vomiting, and headaches. He has no significant medical history. His parents deny recent trauma or recent travel. A magnetic resonance imaging (MRI) scan of the brain shows a tumor in the middle of the cerebellum with mild hydrocephalus. The most likely diagnosis is
   a. Schistosomiasis
   b. Melanoma
   c. Medulloblastoma
   d. Hygroma

17. A patient in the ER is noted to have right-upper quadrant tenderness, a temperature of 102.1° F, and jaundice. This patient most likely has which one of the following conditions?
   a. Ascending cholangitis
   b. Acute appendicitis
   c. Choledocholithiasis
   d. Acute pyelonephritis

18. You have been evaluating a young woman in the office for amenorrhea of eight weeks' duration. Her urine pregnancy test is positive. During the pelvic examination, you notice a bluish discoloration on the vaginal mucosa. Based on her lab findings and physical examination, the name for this bluish discoloration is called
   a. Levine's sign
   b. Kerning's sign
   c. Chadwick's sign
   d. Obturator sign

19. A 58-year-old male comes to the ER with a painful, red, swollen big toe. He has a known history of gout. Based on his past medical history and your examination findings, your first-line treatment would be
   a. Colchicine
   b. Zyloprim
   c. Tetracycline
   d. Amantadine

20. You suspect a patient has benign positional vertigo. Which of the following maneuvers may help aid in your diagnosis?
   a. Dix–Hallpike test
   b. Electroencephalogram (EEG)
   c. Transcranial Doppler ultrasound (TCD)
   d. Phalen's maneuver

21. A 10-year-old child is brought to your office. On physical examination, she is short in stature, has a short wide neck, broad forehead and tongue, and small ears. She has a medical history of mild cognitive and cardiac defects. Which of the following chromosomal defects is most likely the cause for her condition?
   a. 13
   b. 21
   c. 23
   d. 24

22. A patient comes to the ER complaining of pain with inspiration, fever, and palpitations. He recently underwent a coronary artery bypass graft two weeks prior. A cardiology consult is called. The cardiologist tells you he noted "electrical alternans" on your patient's electrocardiogram (EKG). Based on the medical history and EKG findings, you diagnose the patient with
   a. Pericardial tamponade
   b Myocardial infarction
   c. Pneumothorax
   d. Heart murmur

23. A patient comes into the ER complaining of dull, constant, left-sided chest pain for the previous six hours. He is diagnosed with an inferior-wall myocardial infarction (MI). What do you expect the electrocardiogram (EKG) and troponin levels to show?
   a. ST depression in leads V1 through V6 and normal troponin
   b. ST elevation in leads I, aVL, V5, and V6 and elevated troponin
   c. ST elevation in leads II, II, and aVF and elevated troponin
   d. ST depression in leads V7, V8, and V9 and normal troponin

24. You are evaluating a 72-year-old man in the ER for dizziness and syncope. An electrocardiogram (EKG) shows an increasingly prolonged PR interval on consecutive beats followed by a dropped QRS complex. Based on the EKG findings, you are most likely to suspect what type of heart block?
    a. First-degree heart block
    b. Second-degree heart block
    c. Third-degree heart block
    d. Asystole

25. Treatment of asymptomatic sinus bradycardia includes
    a. Continuous telemetry monitoring
    b. Atropine
    c. Epinephrine
    d. Transcutaneous pacing

26. Which of the following is NOT a characteristic of Beck's triad?
    a. Distended jugular veins
    b. Hypotension
    c. Muffled heart sounds
    d. Hypertension

27. All of the following may trigger an asthma attack EXCEPT
    a. Sinusitis
    b. Allergies
    c. Warm air
    d. Smoke

28. Which of the following cells release insulin?
    a. Alpha cells
    b. Beta cells
    c. Gamma cells
    d. Delta cells

29. Which of the following is NOT a complication of diabetes mellitus?
    a. Atherosclerosis
    b. Renal insufficiency
    c. Neuropathy
    d. Hypotension

30. All of the following medications are used to treat *Helicobacter pylori* (*H. pylori*) infections EXCEPT
    a. Clarithromycin, metronidazole, esomeprazole
    b. Amoxicillin, tetracycline, omeprazole
    c. Omeprazole, metronidazole, amoxicillin
    d. Pantoprazole, esomeprazole, clarithromycin

31. All of the following are true about peptic ulcers EXCEPT
    a. Obesity is a major risk factor
    b. It is most commonly caused by *H. pylori*
    c. It can be diagnosed with a stool antigen test
    d. Symptoms are exacerbated by the use of nonsteroidal anti-inflammatory drugs (NSAIDs)

32. In Parkinson's disease, the deterioration of which neurotransmitter is primarily responsible for its symptoms?
    a. Norepinephrine
    b. Epinephrine
    c. Serotonin
    d. Dopamine

33. A person who is diagnosed with Parkinson's disease would have damaged neurons in what area of the brain?
    a. Hippocampus
    b. Pituitary
    c. Substantia nigra
    d. Medulla oblongata

34. Which of the following is most likely associated with left bundle branch block?
    a. Pulmonary embolus
    b. Mitral valve prolapse
    c. Severe aortic valve disease
    d. Pericardial tamponade

35. A 26-year-old female is hospitalized for sickle-cell crisis. Upon admission, she was also found to have a right-lower extremity deep venous thrombus. While examining the patient, you notice that her oxygen saturation on room air drops to 89%, her heart rate is 122, and her respirations are 35 breaths per minute. She is short of breath and complaining of chest pain. Her arterial blood gas (ABG) is normal, and her electrocardiogram (EKG) shows sinus tachycardia. After administering supplemental oxygen, what is your next course of action?
    a. Order a troponin level and wait for the results
    b. Order a computed tomography (CT) angiogram of the chest
    c. Order a CT of the chest without contrast
    d. Repeat the ABG in one hour

36. Which of the following is NOT part of the tetralogy of Fallot?
    a. Atrial septal defect
    b. Narrowing of the pulmonary outflow tract
    c. Right ventricular hypertrophy
    d. Overriding aorta

37. Which of the following is the most common congenital heart defect?
    a. Ventricular septal defect
    b. Tricuspid atresia
    c. Aortic stenosis
    d. Tetralogy of Fallot

38. What is the most common side effect seen with the use of angiotensin-converting enzyme (ACE) inhibitors?
    a. Liver failure
    b. Hypotension
    c. Erectile dysfunction
    d. Cough

39. Which of the following is a gram-positive cocci and is frequently the cause of common skin infections and abscesses?
    a. *Haemophilus influenzae*
    b. *Streptococcus pneumoniae*
    c. *Staphylococcus aureus*
    d. *Staphylococcus pseudintermedius*

40. Which of the following is a treatment for Addison's disease?
    a. Insulin
    b. Somatropin
    c. Synthroid
    d. Cortisol

41. Which of the following is NOT a complication in patients who have chronic obstructive pulmonary disease (COPD)?
    a. Cor pulmonale
    b. Myocardial infarction
    c. Hypotension
    d. Pneumonia

42. Parents bring their toddler into your office. They've noticed that their daughter has had delayed growth, poor weight gain, clay-colored stools, and frequent episodes of pneumonia. You order a sweat chloride test. If the result is positive, what is the most likely diagnosis?
    a. Pneumonia
    b. Cystic fibrosis
    c. Bronchitis
    d. Respiratory syncytial virus

43. Which of the following is TRUE regarding sickle-cell anemia?
    a. It is an autosomal-dominant disease
    b. Heterozygotes are usually asymptomatic
    c. It is due to a defective chromosome 18
    d. It increases your risk of diabetes

44. A 41-year-old female presents to the office with dysuria, frequency, urgency, and lower abdominal discomfort. She denies having fever, chills, back pain, vaginal discharge, nausea, or vomiting. She is in a monogamous relationship and has no history of sexually transmitted diseases. A urine pregnancy test is negative. The urinalysis is positive for leukocytes, bacteria, and nitrites. She has no drug allergies. What is the next step in your medical management?
    a. Prescribe ceftriaxone 250 mg IM x 1 dose
    b. Prescribe azithromycin 1 gm po x 1 dose
    c. Prescribe Augmentin 875 mg po BID x 7 days
    d. Prescribe ciprofloxacin 500 mg po BID x 7 days

45. A 27-year-old patient who is 17 weeks pregnant is diagnosed with a urinary tract infection. She has no drug allergies. What would be your first-choice antibiotic?
    a. Macrobid
    b. Bactrim
    c. Ciprofloxacin
    d. Moxifloxacin

46. A 26-year-old female is seen in your office and diagnosed with chlamydia. This is her fifth sexually transmitted disease in two years. Which of the following interventions in NOT appropriate?
a. Advise her to not tell her partners; they may shun her if they know
b. Counsel her on the use of condoms and other safe-sex measures
c. Treat her with ceftriaxone and azithromycin
d. Order a pregnancy test

47. An 18-year-old male comes to your clinic with a history of periods of "elation and energy" following periods of "sadness and anxiety." He denies suicidal ideation, phobias, new stress or recent trauma, and hallucinations. The physical examination is normal, and the patient is neurologically intact. He has no other significant past medical history. What would be the most likely diagnosis?
a. Dysthymic disorder
b. Bipolar disorder
c. Posttraumatic stress disorder
d. Adjustment disorder

48. A patient recently diagnosed and treated for a urinary tract infection by her primary care doctor now presents to the ER with bright-orange urine of two days' duration. Her urinary tract infection (UTI) symptoms are improved. She cannot recall the medications she was prescribed, but she notes that her symptoms started after taking the medications. She denies allergies to medications, recent travel, or eating new food. Which of the following is most likely the cause for her symptom?
a. Pilocarpine
b. Percodan
c. Pepcid
d. Pyridium

49. A woman comes to your clinic for advice on how to help prevent kidney stone infections. Which of the following is the best advice you would give her?
a. Increase fluid intake, increase carbohydrate intake
b. Decrease fluid intake, increase calcium intake
c. Increase fluid intake, limit calcium intake
d. Decrease fluid intake, decrease protein intake

50. A 32-year-old woman comes to your office complaining of a several-week history of unexplained sadness and anxiety. She no longer enjoys engaging in her extracurricular activities. She denies traumatic events, phobia, hallucinations, or suicidal ideation. She has no significant past medical history. She's never had these symptoms before. Which of the following medications may be beneficial for your patient?
a. Levothyroxine
b. Escitalopram
c. Amiodarone
d. Haloperidol

51. A 14-year-old female patient is brought to your office by her parents with complaints of heavy menses, easy bruising, and recurrent nosebleeds. Her mother notes that she has similar but milder symptoms. Her hemoglobin is 9.8. Her blood work shows that she has a factor VIII clotting deficiency. Which of the following is the most likely diagnosis?
a. Von Willebrand disease
b. Thalassemia
c. Hemophilia
d. Myeloma

52. A 52-year-old male is brought to the ER after falling 10 feet from a ladder and landing on his buttocks. He notes mild pain but has the feeling of "pins and needles" going down both of his lower extremities. He is also complaining of feeling like he has to urinate but is not able to do so. On physical examination, he has decreased lower extremity reflexes, decreased motor strength, and decreased rectal tone. What is the most likely diagnosis?
    a. Fibromyalgia
    b. Greenstick fracture
    c. Cauda equina syndrome
    d. Kyphosis

53. A 13-year-old child is brought to your office complaining of a several-week history of left hip and knee pain. His parent notices that he has been walking with a progressive limp. The child denies trauma or strenuous activity. He has no significant medical problems. On physical examination, you notice that his left leg is slightly shorter than his right. His joints are not swollen or painful. What is the most likely diagnosis?
    a. Developmental dysplasia of the hip
    b. Paget's disease
    c. Slipped capital femoral epiphysis
    d. Osteitis pubis

54. A 66-year-old patient presents to your clinic with progressive bowing of her left femur and tibia as well as pelvis for several months. She notes that she has had two spontaneous leg fractures in the past four months. Her only medical issues are diabetes and gout; she is compliant with her medication regimens. On physical examination, she has notable pelvic enlargement on the left side only. She has bowing of the left leg. Her joints are painful, but they are not red or swollen. Her blood work shows that her serum alkaline phosphatase is elevated. Her computed tomography (CT) scan shows multiple bony deformities on her pelvis and left leg. Based on her lab findings and medical history, which of the following medications would NOT be helpful in treating this patient?
    a. Nonsteroidal anti-inflammatory drugs (NSAIDs)
    b. Calcitonin
    c. Fosamax
    d. Colchicine

55. A 55-year-old female presents to the ER with painless vision loss from her right eye of 30 minutes' duration. She denies photophobia, headache, nausea, vomiting, visual disturbances prior to the vision loss, trauma, or periorbital pain. She has a known history of uncontrolled hypertension and transient ischemic attacks. What is the most likely diagnosis?
    a. Acute angle closure glaucoma
    b. Retinal artery occlusion
    c. Conjunctivitis
    d. Retinal detachment

56. A parent brings her five-year-old daughter into the ER for worsening sore throat, fever, and respiratory distress. The child's oral temperature is 102.5° F. She is drooling and unable to open her mouth. You suspect epiglottitis. Which of the following would NOT be your next course of action?
    a. Administer IV penicillin immediately
    b. Direct visualization of the oropharynx with a tongue depressor
    c. Call a stat ear, nose, and throat (ENT) consultation
    d. Order a lateral cervical spine x ray

57. The most common bacterial pathogen of otitis externa is
   a. *Haemophilus influenzae*
   b. *Pseudomonas aeruginosa*
   c. *Aspergillus*
   d. *Staphylococcus aureus*

58. A 12-year-old child comes to the office with right-sided ear pain, purulent otorrhea, and a fever of 100.5° F. Her father notes that she just returned from a beach vacation, where she spent the majority of her time in the ocean. On physical examination, palpation of her tragus produces pain. Based on her medical history and physical examination, what is your next step?
   a. Stat ear, nose, and throat (ENT) consult
   b. Ofloxacin eardrops
   c. Clindamycin po
   d. Computed tomography (CT) scan

59. A 58-year-old male comes to the office with intermittent vertigo, nausea, tinnitus, and hearing loss. His hearing loss only occurs with the acute vertigo attacks and then returns to baseline. His symptoms started after he had gotten better from a cold about four weeks ago. He notes that although these symptoms are persistent, they are starting to improve. This patient has no significant past medical history. His physical examination is normal. Based on his examination and his medical history, what is the most likely diagnosis?
   a. Labyrinthitis
   b. Ménière's disease
   c. Mastoiditis
   d. Otitis media

60. A 69-year-old male presents to your office with difficulty urinating. He complains of urinary frequency, but decreased urine output. His prostate-specific antigen (PSA) is slightly elevated. On digital rectal examination, he has an enlarged prostate, but no masses or nodules. His urinalysis is normal. What medication would you prescribe for this patient?
   a. Terbinafine
   b. Tegretol
   c. Tramadol
   d. Tamsulosin

61. A female patient has been diagnosed with gestational diabetes, but the diabetes is not controllable by dietary modifications. What is your first step in her medical management?
   a. Start Novolin
   b. Start glyburide
   c. Start pioglitazone
   d. Start glimepiride

62. A patient comes to your clinic, concerned because his brother has just been diagnosed with type 2 diabetes. His father and paternal grandmother were also diabetics. His fasting blood sugar is 98, and his hemoglobin A1C is 5.2. What is the next step in the management of this patient?
   a. Recheck his hemoglobin A1C in a week
   b. Recommend a low-sugar diet and exercise
   c. Start Lantus and metformin
   d. Start metformin only

63. A 35-year-old woman comes to your office for her annual wellness visit. Her examination and vital signs are normal. She has no significant past medical history. She states that her father was diagnosed with colon cancer when he was 48 years old. At what time should this patient get her first colonoscopy?
    a. This year
    b. At 38 years old
    c. At 48 years old
    d. At 50 years old

64. A mother brings her unvaccinated child to the ER with a deep whooping cough. The child is diagnosed with pertussis. Which medication can you prescribe to the mother to help prevent her child from spreading the illness to others?
    a. Augmentin
    b. Clindamycin
    c. Erythromycin
    d. Guaifenesin

65. A father brings in his three-year-old son to the ER with a "barking" cough, runny nose, and a fever of 100.5° F. The child attends day care. He has no other significant past medical history. On physical examination, he is noted to have the aforementioned cough, clear rhinorrhea, and mild wheezing bilaterally. He is not in any acute respiratory distress. Based on his physical examination and medical history, what is the most likely diagnosis?
    a. Pneumonia
    b. Cystic fibrosis
    c. Respiratory syncytial virus (RSV)
    d. Asthma

66. A 26-year-old man is rushed to the emergency room with chest pain and shortness of breath that developed suddenly. A family member notes that he has smoked a half a pack of cigarettes per day for five years, but he has no other known medical problems. On physical examination, there is no evidence of trauma. He has normal breath sounds on the left but decreased breath sounds on the right. A chest x-ray shows lung markings on the left, but not on the right. Based on his past medical history, presentation, and x-ray, what is the most likely diagnosis?
    a. Pneumonia
    b. Secondary pneumothorax
    c. Pulmonary carcinoma
    d. Spontaneous pneumothorax

67. A 30-year-old man comes to the ER with a two-week history of hemoptysis, fever, and chills. He has no significant past medical history. A chest x-ray shows multiple cavitary lesions. Based on his chest x-ray and his symptoms, what is your diagnosis?
    a. Bronchitis
    b. Tuberculosis
    c. Pneumothorax
    d. Lung cancer

68. A 19-year-old patient comes to your clinic complaining of recurrent nasal congestion. She states that her primary care doctor gave her a nasal spray. It helped her symptoms for the first three days. She continued to use it for another four days, and the nasal congestion reoccurred. Which of the following medications are most likely to blame for her symptoms?
    a. Oxymetazoline hydrochloride
    b. Benzonatate
    c. Ofloxacin
    d. Guaifenesin

69. A 58-year-old male patient comes to your office concerned because he has a family history of heart disease and would like to be worked up. His father and older brother died of heart attacks. This patient's LDL is 150. His weight, vital signs, stress test, two-dimensional echocardiogram, and electrocardiogram (EKG) are normal. He has no significant past medical history. What medications would you recommend for this patient?
    a. A baby aspirin and amlodipine
    b. Amlodipine and simvastatin
    c. A baby aspirin and metoprolol
    d. A baby aspirin and simvastatin

70. A mother brings her one-month-old son into your office for evaluation. He has had poor weight gain, even though he seems to be constantly hungry. She states that the child has an episode of projectile vomiting after almost every feeding. You notice that the child's abdomen is distended, and you palpate an olive-shaped mass in the epigastrium. Based on the medical history and physical examination, what is the most likely diagnosis?
    a. Gastroesophageal reflux disease (GERD)
    b. Gastritis
    c. Pyloric stenosis
    d. Mallory–Weiss tear

71. A 69-year-old male with a history of alcohol abuse comes to the ER after having an episode of hematemesis following binge drinking. Recently he's also been noticing black, tarry stools. He states that he's vomited blood on several occasions, but these episodes have been becoming more frequent. He denies unintentional weight loss or gain, abdominal pain, diarrhea, fever, recent illness, history of bleeding disorders, or lymphadenopathy. His stool guaiac is positive. His physical examination is normal. He currently feels fine. Based on his medical history and physical examination, what is the most likely diagnosis?
    a. Celiac sprue
    b. Whipple's disease
    c. Mallory–Weiss tear
    d. Pyloric stenosis

72. A mother brings her toddler into the office for an evaluation. The mother notes that the child's right eye deviates toward her nose. The child has had this condition since she was an infant. Her pupils are equal and reactive. Based on her medical history and physical examination, what is the most likely diagnosis?
    a. Exotropia
    b. Hypertropia
    c. Esotropia
    d. Hypotropia

73. A father brings his child to the ER noting a two-day history of red eyes, low-grade fever, and crusting of the eyelids and eyelashes. He states that many of her classmates have similar symptoms. On physical examination, the child has erythematous conjunctiva bilaterally with golden crusts on her eyelids and lashes. The child denies pain. The child's pupils are equal and reactive, and her vision is normal. She has no medical problems. Based on her medical history and physical examination findings, what is the most likely diagnosis?
    a. Allergic conjunctivitis
    b. Bacterial conjunctivitis
    c. Viral conjunctivitis
    d. Dacryoadenitis

74. A six-year-old patient comes to the ER and is diagnosed with bacterial conjunctivitis. She has no past medical history and is up to date on all of her vaccinations. What is the next step in your medical management?
    a. Erythromycin
    b. Trifluridine
    c. Ciprofloxacin
    d. Famciclovir

75. A 68-year-old female newly diagnosed with hyperlipidemia comes to the ER after she noticed her entire body turning a reddish color and associated mild itching. She was just started on a new medication for her high cholesterol last week, but she cannot remember the name. She denies recent travel, new soaps or detergents, new foods, chest pain, shortness of breath, or palpitations. Other than her generalized flushing and pruritus, her physical examination seems normal. What medication has most likely caused her symptoms?
    a. Atorvastatin
    b. Rosuvastatin
    c. Simvastatin
    d. Niacin

76. A 58-year-old man presents to the ER with a temperature of 101.5° F, productive cough with yellow sputum, shaking chills, and mild dyspnea for the past two days. His oxygen saturation is 98% on room air. A chest x-ray shows an infiltrate on the lower left lobe. He has no significant past medical history. What is the next step in your medical management?
    a. Start po antibiotics and discharge home
    b. Order a computed tomography (CT) scan of the chest
    c. Admit to the hospital and start intravenous (IV) antibiotics
    d. Obtain an arterial blood gas (ABG)

77. A patient with hyperlipidemia that you have recently placed on niacin develops mild generalized flushing and pruritus. What would NOT be the next step in your medical management?
    a. Discontinue the medication immediately
    b. Continue the medication and adjust the dosage
    c. Give Decadron and Benadryl for symptomatic relief
    d. Have the patient take nonsteroidal anti-inflammatory drugs (NSAIDs) prior to niacin dose

78. A father brings his two-year-old son to the ER for a three-day history of runny nose, a temperature of 100.5° F, and nasal congestion. Today, the child developed a barking cough. The child is not in any respiratory distress, and his appetite, fluid intake, and urinary output have all been normal. What is the next step in your medical management?
    a. Discharge home, recommend fluids and humidified air
    b. Discharge home with oral steroids only
    c. Discharge home with oral steroids and oral antibiotics
    d. Discharge home with oral antibiotics only

79. An HIV-positive patient is diagnosed with *Pneumocystis* pneumonia. What is the first-line treatment?
    a. Gentamicin
    b. Trimethoprim-sulfamethoxazole
    c. Augmentin
    d. Corticosteroids

80. A newborn is diagnosed with phenylketonuria (PKU). What can you do as a health-care provider to minimize the sequelae of this disease?
    a. Prescribe Ritalin
    b. Prescribe Dilantin
    c. Advise routine blood work
    d. Advise parents about dietary restrictions

81. What is the most effective way to prevent the spread of communicable diseases?
    a. Maintaining a sterile environment
    b. Wearing gloves
    c. Hand washing
    d. Wearing a face mask while working with sick patients

82. Which of the following is NOT a way to prevent listeriosis?
    a. Thoroughly rinse raw produce
    b. Refrain from ingesting unpasteurized milk
    c. Limit intake of processed meats during pregnancy
    d. Refrain from eating fish or seafood during pregnancy

83. What is the most effective way to prevent rabies infection?
    a. Immediately obtaining the rabies vaccine
    b. Immediately cleansing the wound
    c. Administering po Augmentin
    d. Administering IV clindamycin

84. Which of the following is NOT a way to treat scabies?
    a. Lotrimin cream
    b. Permethrin cream
    c. Washing linens and clothing in hot water
    d. Avoiding contact with infected people

- 16 -

85. A 24-year-old man presents to the ER with worsening left-sided abdominal pain radiating to the back, temperature of 100.5° F, shaking chills, nausea, and vomiting of three days' duration. On physical examination, he has mild left-epigastric pain with moderate left-sided costovertebral angle tenderness. His urinalysis is positive for red blood cells only. His white blood cell (WBC) count is 16,000. His basic metabolic panel, amylase, lipase, and liver function tests are normal. Based on his medical history, physical examination, and lab results, what is the most likely diagnosis?
    a. Hepatitis
    b. Cholecystitis
    c. Appendicitis
    d. Nephrolithiasis

86. Which of the following is the least likely to cause a cardiac arrest?
    a. Hyperkalemia
    b. Hypervolemia
    c. Hypokalemia
    d. Hypovolemia

87. An 11-year-old male is brought to the ER by his mother with a one-day history of sudden, right-sided abdominal pain, nausea, and vomiting. These symptoms are not related to food intake. There is no history of trauma, recent travel, ingesting raw or rare foods, or diarrhea. His only medical problem is asthma. During his physical examination, he cries out in pain while you gently shake the bed. He displays moderate discomfort when you flex his right leg at his hip and his knee. What is the most likely diagnosis based on his medical history and examination findings?
    a. Nephrolithiasis
    b. Appendicitis
    c. Cholecystitis
    d. Hepatitis

88. A mother brings her 16-year-old daughter to the ER for a two-day history of fever, nausea, vomiting, photophobia, and severe constant generalized headache. There is no history of trauma. The child has no significant past medical history. During her physical examination, she flexes her hip and knee when you flex her neck. Based on her presenting symptoms and her examination, what is the most likely diagnosis?
    a. Subarachnoid hemorrhage
    b. Migraines
    c. Vestibulocerebellar syndrome
    d. Meningitis

89. A 56-year-old man comes to the ER with dull, nonradiating left-sided chest pain, nausea, and vomiting for the past four hours. The chest pain is not related to activity. He denies a history of similar symptoms. You notice that his blood pressure is 80/45 and that his electrocardiogram (EKG) shows sinus tachycardia with a rate of 123. His oxygen saturation is 99% on room air. During his physical examination, you notice that his neck veins are bulging. Auscultation of his heart reveals quiet systolic and diastolic sounds. His breath sounds are coarse bilaterally. Based on his symptoms and physical examination, what is the most likely diagnosis?
    a. Pericardial tamponade
    b. Pneumothorax
    c. Aortic dissection
    d. Stable angina

90. A patient's electrocardiogram (EKG) shows a prolonged PR interval that regularly precedes a QRS complex. The PR interval remains unchanged. What is the most likely diagnosis based on the EKG findings?

    a. First-degree heart block
    b. Second-degree heart block (Mobitz type I)
    c. Second-degree heart block (Mobitz type II)
    d. Third-degree heart block

91. A 19-year-old female patient comes to your office with her parent, who is concerned about the deterioration of her daughter's health over the past several months. The daughter admits to being depressed. Her vital signs and weight are normal. On physical examination, you notice that she has multiple cavities and gingivitis. The patient admits that she sometimes forces herself to vomit after meals to help control her weight. Based on her medical history and physical, what is the most likely diagnosis?

    a. Anorexia nervosa
    b. Panic disorder
    c. Bulimia nervosa
    d. Dysthymic disorder

92. A 28-year-old male patient is brought to your clinic by his brother, who states that his brother's behavior is becoming increasingly erratic. He has intermittent episodes of agitation. The patient has been stating that he has been seeing and talking to his father, even though his father passed away five years ago. The patient also has been having trouble concentrating and often skips from different topics during a conversation in a few minutes. The patient confides in you that his brother is "part of a conspiracy to lock him away." The patient's labs are all normal and so are his vital signs. His physical examination is normal as well. A computed tomography (CT) scan of the brain shows no acute abnormalities. Based on his medical history, physical examination, and labs, what is the next step in your management?

    a. Start haloperidol and a psychiatry referral
    b. Start paroxetine and a psychiatry referral
    c. Start escitalopram and a psychiatry referral
    d. Start zolpidem and a psychiatry referral

93. Parents bring their one-month-old son to your clinic for failure to thrive, pallor, dark urine, and jaundice since birth. His vital signs are normal. His complete blood count (CBC) and iron panel show hemolytic anemia. His platelets, white blood cell (WBC) count, liver function tests, amylase, and lipase are normal. On physical examination, the child is mildly lethargic but easily aroused. You notice that he has jaundice. Based on his past medical history, physical examination, and labs, what is the most likely diagnosis?

    a. Leukocytosis
    b. Thrombocytopenia
    c. Glucose-6-phosphate dehydrogenase (G6PD) deficiency
    d. Von Willebrand disease

94. One of your pediatric patients has just been diagnosed with thalassemia major. The parents ask you what they can do to limit the severity of symptoms and improve their child's quality of life. What suggestions do you give them?

    a. Blood transfusions and iron supplements
    b. Limit folate and iron intake
    c. Folate supplements and regular blood transfusions
    d. Avoid nonsteroidal anti-inflammatory drugs (NSAIDs), legumes, and henna

95. A 24-year-old female who is twenty-six weeks pregnant comes to the ER for sudden onset of bright-red, painless vaginal bleeding. She has no medical problems; she does not smoke, drink, or use drugs, and hasn't had any prior complications during this pregnancy. Other than the vaginal bleeding, she does not have any symptoms. Her complete blood count (CBC) is normal. An ultrasound reveals that the placenta is touching the top of the cervix. What is the most likely diagnosis based on her symptoms, labs, and ultrasound findings?
    a. Placental abruption (abruptio placentae)
    b. Premature rupture of membranes
    c. Dystocia
    d. Placenta previa

96. A 35-year-old woman who is six weeks pregnant comes to the ER for mild vaginal bleeding and mild low-back pain. Her transvaginal ultrasound is negative for an intrauterine pregnancy. Her serum beta human chorionic gonadotropin (HCG) is normal. What is the next step in your medical management?
    a. Stat surgical consult for laparoscopy
    b. Repeat her beta HCG and ultrasound in two days
    c. Discharge home and recommend bed rest
    d. Administer methotrexate

97. A child has been recently diagnosed with impetigo. Which of the following recommendations would NOT prevent the spread of the infection?
    a. You may touch the skin lesions once antibiotics have been started
    b. Wash hands thoroughly after touching the patient
    c. Clean all clothes and bed linens in hot water
    d. Do not share personal care items with the patient

98. You diagnose a patient with tinea corporis. Which of the following medications would treat this condition?
    a. Erythromycin
    b. Ketoconazole
    c. Mupirocin
    d. Metronidazole

99. A father brings his 13-year-old son to the ER. He states that the foreskin of his son's penis is "stuck." The penis is mildly swollen and erythematous. The testes are normal. Upon physical examination, you note that the foreskin cannot be reduced. The most likely diagnosis is
    a. Phimosis
    b. Hydrocele
    c. Paraphimosis
    d. Cryptorchidism

100. A two-month-old male is brought to your clinic for a routine wellness examination. During his physical examination, you notice that you cannot palpate his left testicle. Your next step in his medical management is to
    a. Recommend a surgical consult for possible orchiopexy
    b. Recommend a computed tomography (CT) scan
    c. Recommend hormone injections
    d. Recommend to monitor the child for now

101. A 22-year-old male comes to your clinic with a painless mass on his right testicle of two weeks' duration. He denies trauma, lymphadenopathy, or prior infection. His complete blood count (CBC) and chemistry are normal. A physical examination reveals a soft, fluctuant, nontender mass. You shine a flashlight at the mass, which transmits light. Based on his medical history and physical examination, what is the most likely diagnosis?
    a. Hydrocele
    b. Testicular torsion
    c. Varicocele
    d. Cryptorchidism

102. A 21-year-old patient in the hospital for sickle-cell crisis is newly diagnosed with a pulmonary embolus. She has no past medical history other than sickle-cell disease. Which of the following would NOT be part of your medical management once the patient's oxygenation status is stabilized?
    a. Surgery consult for an inferior vena cava (IVC) filter
    b. Start heparin infusion
    c. Administer analgesics for the chest pain
    d. Repeat D-dimer in one week

103. A 30-year-old patient in your clinic tells you that he seems to get the flu every year. Other than smoking a half a pack of cigarettes per day for the past five years, he is healthy. He asks you how he can avoid contracting the flu this year. Which of the following is NOT part of your recommendations?
    a. Frequent hand washing while at work or at a public venue
    b. Obtaining the influenza vaccine in the fall
    c. Avoid the influenza vaccine because he is not in a high-risk group
    d. Decrease his tobacco use

104. All of the following medications will treat atrial fibrillation EXCEPT?
    a. Lanoxin
    b. Furosemide
    c. Metoprolol
    d. Warfarin

105. A patient visits your office for his annual wellness examination. He tells you he had recently become ill after visiting the southwest part of the United States. He had painful red lumps on his lower legs, blood-tinged sputum, loss of appetite, fever, night sweats, and headache. The symptoms spontaneously resolved on their own without treatment. A doctor who saw him in the ER while he was in the southwest said he had valley fever. The patient's vital signs and physical examination are normal. He has no past medical history. Based on his symptoms and medical history, what illness did your patient most likely have?
    a. *Pneumocystis* pneumonia
    b. Tuberculosis
    c. Respiratory syncytial virus (RSV)
    d. Coccidioidomycosis

106. Which of the following can make a definitive diagnosis of ventricular septal defect?
    a. Echocardiogram
    b. Chest x ray
    c. Electrocardiogram (EKG)
    d. Auscultation with a stethoscope

107. A mother brings in her six-year-old daughter to the ER for syncope, worsening chest pain, shortness of breath, and dizziness. The mother notes that her daughter always seems to have cold legs. The child has a past medical history of Turner syndrome. A chest x-ray shows cardiomegaly. A cardiologist is called, who notes the figure 3 sign on the chest x-ray. Based on the medical history, presentation, and imaging findings, what is the most likely diagnosis?
   a. Tetralogy of Fallot
   b. Coarctation of the aorta
   c. Hypoplastic left heart syndrome
   d. Tricuspid atresia

108. A 56-year-old female patient with a history of alcohol abuse presents to the ER with dizziness, chest pain, palpitations, and syncope. A cardiologist viewing her electrocardiogram (EKG) mentions that the QRS complex twists around the isoelectric baseline. What cardiac arrhythmia is the cardiologist most likely describing?
   a. Bundle branch block
   b. Sick sinus syndrome
   c. Torsades de pointes
   d. Atrial fibrillation

109. A 24-year-old woman presents to your clinic with persistent chest pain and shortness of breath, which commonly occur at rest. Exercise does not induce her symptoms. She has been to the ER several times with these symptoms. Her electrocardiogram (EKG), troponin level, chest x ray, and two-dimensional echocardiogram are all normal. She had a prior cardiac catheterization one year ago, which was negative. Her physical examination is normal; palpation of her chest wall does not reproduce symptoms. She has no medical problems. She admits to smoking a pack of cigarettes a day for five years. What is the most likely diagnosis?
   a. Prinzmetal's angina
   b. Unstable angina
   c. Stable angina
   d. Costochondritis

110. Which of the following can be the cause of syndrome of inappropriate antidiuretic hormone (SIADH)?
   a. Squamous-cell carcinoma
   b. Large-cell carcinoma
   c. Adenocarcinoma
   d. Small-cell carcinoma

111. A patient presents to the ER with suspected infective endocarditis. Which of the following tests would be the least helpful diagnostic aid?
   a. Computed tomography (CT) scan of the chest
   b. Echocardiogram
   c. Chest x-ray
   d. Blood cultures

112. A patient has come to your clinic for multiple visits over the past several weeks with a persistently borderline elevated blood pressure. Today it is 138/88. He has no family history of hypertension. He smokes less than a half a pack of cigarettes per day, but otherwise he has no medical problems. Which of the following would be recommendations to help him lower his blood pressure without medications?
    a. Limit tobacco use, increase sodium intake, increase physical activity
    b. Decrease stress, increase tobacco use, increase physical activity
    c. Decrease sodium intake, increase physical activity, limit tobacco use
    d. Limit tobacco use, decrease sodium intake, decrease physical activity

113. You are evaluating a 52-year-old female patient in your office for the first time. During auscultation of her heart, you hear a midsystolic click. The murmur gets louder when she stands up. The patient informs you that she has a known history of a heart murmur. She denies chest pain, dyspnea, dizziness, and palpitations. Her electrocardiogram (EKG) is normal. Her echocardiogram reveals a mitral valve that does not fully close. What is your next step in her medical management?
    a. Recommend cardiology referral for possible catheterization
    b. Order a computed tomography (CT) scan of the chest
    c. Monitor for now; no intervention is needed
    d. Order a repeat EKG in one month

114. A 61-year-old male presents to the ER with the sudden onset of dull, throbbing, left-sided chest pain radiating to his jaw and back, nausea, vomiting, and diaphoresis. An electrocardiogram (EKG) shows an inferior wall non-ST segment elevation myocardial infarction (NSTEMI). His vital signs are as follows: BP, 165/98; pulse, 92 beats per minute; pulse oximetry, 93% on room air; and respirations, 26 per minute. The patient is awake and alert, but in moderate pain. After administering oxygen, which of the following would be the next step in your medical management?
    a. Order metoprolol, morphine, and clopidogrel
    b. Order aspirin, metoprolol, and nitroglycerin
    c. Order an echocardiogram and troponin level
    d. Order metoprolol, aspirin, and clopidogrel

115. A 68-year-old male comes to the ER after having an episode of left-sided chest pain radiating to his left arm for 10 minutes. He had been mowing his lawn when the chest pain occurred. It resolved about 5 minutes after he sat down to rest. He states that he often gets similar symptoms during physical activity. The symptoms resolve with rest. He currently has no medical complaints. His past medical history includes hyperlipidemia and obesity. His physical examination is normal. His vital signs are as follows: BP, 155/91; pulse, 88 beats per minute, pulse oximetry, 98% on room air; and respirations, 16 per minute. Based on his past medical history and physical examination, what is the most likely diagnosis?
    a. Stable angina
    b. Prinzmetal's angina
    c. Variant angina
    d. Aortic aneurysm

116. A 77-year-old female patient comes to your clinic complaining of worsening vision for the past month. She notes that the center of her vision has been deteriorating. It has become incredibly difficult for her to read. Her peripheral vision remains intact. She denies the presence of floaters or flashes of light, photophobia, headache, nausea, vomiting, or trauma. Her past medical history includes osteoarthritis and osteoporosis. She denies trauma or recent illness. What is the most likely diagnosis?
   a. Optic neuritis
   b. Macular degeneration
   c. Glaucoma
   d. Retinal artery occlusion

117. A 42-year-old female comes to the ER for right-sided tinnitus, worsening ataxia, right-sided hearing loss, dizziness, and headache of one month's duration. She denies trauma or recent illness. She has no significant past medical history. The symptoms are not exacerbated or alleviated by motion. Her physical examination is normal. What is the next step in your medical management?
   a. Order an electromyography
   b. Order an ear, nose, and throat (ENT) consult
   c. Perform the Dix–Hallpike maneuver
   d. Order a magnetic resonance imaging (MRI) scan of the brain

118. A four-year-old female child is brought in for persistent coughing. Prior to the coughing episode, the child had been seen playing with a toy car. The toy car cannot be found. The child's oxygen saturation on room air is 91%. Upon physical examination, you do not see an object in the child's oropharynx. Her lungs are diminished on the right. The child has stridor. After administering oxygen, what is the next step in your medical management?
   a. Order stat chest x-ray
   b. Perform a finger sweep to see if you can remove the object
   c. Administer nebulizer treatment
   d. Order a stat bronchoscopy

119. A 76-year-old female comes to the ER with nonproductive cough, chest pain with inspiration, and shortness of breath of two days' duration. Her vital signs are as follows: BP, 144/72; respirations, 25 per minute; pulse, 101 beats per minute; and oxygen saturation on room air, 93%. On physical examination, she has diminished breath sounds on the right side. She has dullness to percussion and decreased tactile fremitus on the right side. She has a known history of tobacco abuse and chronic obstructive pulmonary disease (COPD). Based on your physical examination, what is the most likely diagnosis?
   a. Asthma
   b. Pleural effusion
   c. Pneumothorax
   d. Influenza

120. A patient comes to your office complaining of progressive knee pain of one month's duration. You suspect a meniscus tear. Which of the following maneuvers would you do to help confirm the diagnosis?
   a. Obturator test
   b. McMurray test
   c. Murphy test
   d McBurney point tenderness

121. You are evaluating an x ray of a patient who fell; it shows a bone fragment separated from the bone. What kind of fracture is this?
  a. Avulsion fracture
  b. Greenstick fracture
  c. Comminuted fracture
  d. Oblique fracture

122. A 65-year-old male comes to your office with worsening cough and dyspnea of two months' duration. He has no other medical problems. He states that he had worked in a coal mine for 30 years, but he has recently retired. His lungs on chest x ray show a honeycomb pattern. Based on your findings, what is the most likely diagnosis?
  a. Pneumoconiosis
  b. Schistosomiasis
  c. Coccidioidomycosis
  d. Tuberculosis

123. A 21-year-old male comes to your office after finding a hard, fixed, painless lump on his testicle. He's never had testicular lesions before. He has no past medical history. You shine a penlight at the lesion; it does not transmit light. Based on your physical examination, what is the most likely diagnosis?
  a. Hydrocele
  b. Testicular carcinoma
  c. Varicocele
  d. Testicular torsion

124. A patient comes to your office complaining of persistent unilateral shoulder pain that started after his wrestling match at school. You suspect a rotator cuff tear. Which of the following tests would you perform to help confirm the diagnosis?
  a. Anterior drawer test
  b. Lachman test
  c. McMurray test
  d. Drop-arm test

125. A mother brings her six-year-old daughter to the ER for left-sided ear pain of three days' duration associated with mild hearing loss, swelling, and fever. She states that her daughter had been recently treated for an inner ear infection one week prior. The child has no ataxia, vertigo, lymphadenopathy, tinnitus, nausea, or vomiting. Her temperature in the ER is 102.1° F. On physical examination, you notice mild displacement of the ear caused by swelling of the posterior ear. Her tympanic membrane is erythematous. Based on her medical history and physical examination, what is the most likely diagnosis?
  a. Acoustic neuroma
  b. Cholesteatoma
  c. Mastoiditis
  d. Ménière's disease

126. A 51-year-old HIV patient presents with fever, headache, nausea, and vomiting. His complete blood count (CBC) shows a leukocytosis with bandemia. A lumbar puncture is performed, and cultures are sent to the lab. His India ink stain is positive. What is the most likely organism causing his meningitis?
  a. *Histoplasma*
  b. *Neisseria*
  c. *Cryptococcus*
  d. *Haemophilus*

- 24 -

127. A five-year-old child is brought to the ER by his father for an acute asthma exacerbation. Which of the following would NOT be a treatment of choice in an acute asthma exacerbation?
   a. Singulair
   b. Xopenex
   c. Ventolin
   d. Proventil

128. A mother brings her toddler into your office for a multitude of symptoms. Her daughter has been developing nausea, vomiting, fever, and abdominal pain for the past several weeks. During the child's physical examination, you notice that the child has a nontender abdominal mass. The patient also has no right iris (aniridia) and has unilateral swelling on one side of her body. The mother states that she has a family history of cancer, but she can't remember what kind. Based on the child's medical history and physical examination, what kind of tumor is most likely responsible for the child's symptoms?
   a. Hodgkin's lymphoma
   b. Lipoma
   c. Wilms' tumor
   d. Kaposi sarcoma

129. A mother gives birth to her baby at 28 weeks of gestation. Immediately after labor, the child goes into respiratory distress. No complications have occurred during the pregnancy prior to labor. The mother has no relevant past medical history. What is the most likely diagnosis for the child's respiratory symptoms?
   a. Respiratory syncytial virus (RSV)
   b. Hyaline membrane disease
   c. *Pneumocystis* pneumonia
   d. Pneumoconiosis

130. A 21-year-old male presents to the ER with right-sided eye pain after being involved in a physical altercation. His right conjunctiva has a medial well-circumscribed erythematous area. His extraocular muscles (EOMs) are intact, and his pupils are equal and reactive. He has no vision loss or periorbital swelling. Based on his medical history and physical examination, what is the most likely diagnosis?
   a. Blepharitis
   b. Hordeolum
   c. Hyphema
   d. Optic neuritis

131. You are examining a patient in the ER for acute alcohol intoxication. He is well known to the ER for his chronic alcoholism. During your physical examination, you notice that he has white patches on his tongue that cannot be scraped off. This condition is called
   a. Leukoplakia
   b. Oral thrush
   c. Parotitis
   d. Gingivostomatitis

132. A cardiologist is examining the chest x ray of a child with a known cyanotic heart defect. He mentions that the child has a "boot-shaped heart." What heart defect does the child most likely have?
   a. Ventricular septal defect
   b. Patent ductus arteriosus
   c. Atrial septal defect
   d. Tetralogy of Fallot

133. A patient presents to your office with various symptoms. Based on the patient's medical history and physical examination, you suspect sarcoidosis. Which of the following tests would you order to confirm the diagnosis?
    a. Computed tomography (CT) scan of the chest
    b. Bronchoscopy with biopsy
    c. Lumbar puncture
    d. Serum phosphorus

134. A 28-year-old female comes to your clinic concerned because she has been developing multiple painful breast lumps over the past several months. They enlarge and shrink in size during the month. During your physical examination, you find multiple bilateral soft, painful breast masses. There is no erythema, skin changes, nipple discharge, or lymphadenopathy. What is the most likely diagnosis?
    a. Breast cancer
    b. Fibroadenoma
    c. Fibrocystic breast disease
    d. Gynecomastia

135. A 26-year-old patient has just been diagnosed with a fibroadenoma via biopsy. What is the next step in your medical management?
    a. Monitor for now; no further intervention is needed
    b. Recommend birth control pills
    c. Repeat biopsy in two months
    d. Recommend surgical consultation for a mastectomy

136. Which of the following is NOT a treatment for active tuberculosis?
    a. Clindamycin
    b. Amikacin
    c. Streptomycin
    d. Ethambutol

137. Which of the following remedies would NOT help alleviate the effects of barotrauma?
    a. Chew gum
    b. Suck on candy
    c. Yawn
    d. Ascend quickly

138. A father brings his one-year-old daughter in for mild respiratory distress of one day's duration. Originally, her symptoms started out like a common cold, but then she developed a noisy, nonproductive cough and low-grade fever. On physical examination, you notice intercostal retractions. Her temperature is 100.5° F; otherwise, her vitals are normal. Based on her medical history and physical examination, what is the most likely diagnosis?
    a. Hyaline membrane disease
    b. Bronchiolitis
    c. Tuberculosis
    d. Cystic fibrosis

139. Which of the following is a first-line treatment for Hashimoto's thyroiditis?
   a. Lantus
   b. Levothyroxine
   c. Lanoxin
   d. Lamisil

140. A 45-year-old man with no history of medical problems has developed worsening, unpredictable mood changes and a decline in cognitive function. He has recently developed an ataxic gait and uncoordinated, jerky body movements. What is the most likely diagnosis?
   a. Tourette syndrome
   b. Guillain–Barré syndrome
   c. Cerebral palsy
   d. Huntington's disease

141. A patient presents with myalgias, fatigue, and diffuse bony pain. Further workup reveals the presence of osteoporosis and nephrolithiasis. What is the most likely diagnosis?
   a. Hyperthyroidism
   b. Hypoparathyroidism
   c. Hyperparathyroidism
   d. Hypothyroidism

142. What is the first-line treatment for a scabies infection?
   a. Permethrin
   b. Olanzapine
   c. Phenergan
   d. Ondansetron

143. A patient with a known history of gout comes to your clinic asking about what he can do to reduce the occurrence of his gout attacks. Which of the following dietary recommendations would you NOT recommend?
   a. Reduce red meat intake
   b. Reduce seafood intake
   c. Reduce calcium intake
   d. Reduce alcohol intake

144. A 25-year-old female is admitted to the hospital for fever of unknown origin. She has a temperature of 102.3° F and is complaining of fever, chills, and diaphoresis. She has a known history of intravenous (IV) drug abuse. The attending physician notes that the patient has Janeway lesions. Based on her medical history and physical examination, the most likely diagnosis is
   a. Pneumonia
   b. Meningitis
   c. Endocarditis
   d. *Clostridium difficile* colitis

145. Which of the following medications would you NOT use in a patient with restrictive cardiomyopathy?
   a. Furosemide
   b. Metoprolol
   c. Aspirin
   d. Epinephrine

146. A patient with *Clostridium difficile* colitis has been experiencing worsening abdominal pain and fever. An abdominal x ray shows colonic distension. What is the most likely diagnosis based on symptoms and x-ray findings?
   a. Ogilvie's syndrome
   b. Toxic megacolon
   c. Intussusception
   d. Hirschsprung's disease

147. A patient with a known history of alcoholism comes to the ER with left-upper quadrant pain radiating to his back for the past day. He's had this pain previously after an alcohol binge, but this episode is much more painful. What is the most likely diagnosis?
   a. Cholangitis
   b. Mallory–Weiss tear
   c. Pancreatitis
   d. Hepatitis

148. Family members bring a 61-year-old man to your office for the first time for a wellness checkup. As they are filling out paperwork, you notice that he has a resting tremor, slow movements, rigidity, and shuffling gait. What is the most likely diagnosis?
   a. Huntington's disease
   b. Alzheimer's dementia
   c. Parkinson's disease
   d. Guillain–Barré syndrome

149. A 42-year-old female with a known history of systemic lupus erythematous comes to your office with a myriad of complaints including unintentional weight gain, increase in body hair, acne, stretch marks, and muscle weakness. She takes prednisone and nonsteroidal anti-inflammatory drugs (NSAIDs) to help control her lupus symptoms. What is the most likely diagnosis?
   a. Cushing's syndrome
   b. Addison's disease
   c. Acromegaly
   d. Hashimoto's disease

150. A 21-year-old female comes to the ER complaining of a blistering rash and facial swelling that started in the morning. She has never had this rash before. She has no significant past medical history. The only medication she is currently taking is penicillin for streptococcal pharyngitis. On physical examination, you notice diffuse dark reddish purple papular rash on her trunk, face, and extremities with extensive blister formation. Her temperature is 99.9° F; otherwise, her vitals are normal. Based on her medical history and physical examination, what is the most likely diagnosis?
   a. Turner syndrome
   b. Stevens–Johnson syndrome
   c. Cushing's syndrome
   d. Guillain–Barré syndrome

151. A mother brings her six-year-old son in for his annual wellness visit. The child has no past medical history. During the examination, his mother states that about three weeks ago, the child had a viral infection. Following the viral infection, she noticed pinpoint reddish-purple dots on his extremities that appeared and spontaneously disappeared. Currently, the child's examination and vital signs are normal. Based on his medical history and physical examination, what was the most likely diagnosis causing his dermal symptoms?
    a. Idiopathic thrombocytopenic purpura
    b. Stevens–Johnson syndrome
    c. Von Willebrand disease
    d. Glucose-6-phosphate dehydrogenase (G6PD) deficiency

152. A couple brings their three-year-old daughter to the ER for worsening cough, fever, and sore throat. The child has no past medical history; however, the parents admit that they did not have their daughter vaccinated. On physical examination, you notice that the child is slightly cyanotic. You also see a grayish-black, tough, fiberlike covering of her oropharynx. Based on her medical history and physical examination, what is the most likely diagnosis?
    a. Cryptococcosis
    b. Shigellosis
    c. Cholera
    d. Diphtheria

153. A mother brings her 16-year-old daughter to the ER complaining of fever, sore throat, lethargy, and swollen cervical lymph glands. The child's temperature is 100.1° F; her other vital signs are normal. The child is mildly lethargic but easily aroused and does not appear to be dehydrated. Her physical examination is essentially normal other than her cervical lymphadenopathy. A monospot test is positive. What is the next step in your medical management?
    a. Prescribe amantadine
    b. Prescribe Augmentin
    c. Recommend computed tomography (CT) scan of the abdomen
    d. Recommend rest and fluids

154. A 71-year-old male comes to your office with a history of multiple, nontraumatic fractures for the past six months. Blood work reveals hypercalcemia and anemia, and his BUN/creatinine are 36/1.7. Urine studies reveal the presence of the Bence Jones protein. What is the most likely diagnosis?
    a. Acute myelogenous leukemia (AML)
    b. Multiple myeloma
    c. Acute lymphocytic leukemia (ALL)
    d. Paget's disease

155. Which of the following would be the LEAST helpful diagnostic test in diagnosing hemolytic anemia?
    a. International normalized ratio (INR)
    b. Coombs' test, direct
    c. Complete blood count (CBC)
    d. Lactate dehydrogenase (LDH) test

156. An infant is born with microcephaly, deafness, chorioretinitis, hepatosplenomegaly, and thrombocytopenia. Which of the following diseases would NOT be a likely cause?
   a. Influenza
   b. Rubella
   c. Toxoplasmosis
   d. Cytomegalovirus

157. A patient is diagnosed with mild iron-deficiency anemia. Which of the following foods would you NOT recommend your patient to increase his iron intake?
   a. Spinach
   b. Eggs
   c. Pasta
   d. Oranges

158. A 45-year-old patient comes to your clinic with an itchy, purplish rash on her wrists and ankle of five days' duration. She's had this rash before, but it usually resolves on its own. Other than the rash, she generally feels well. She has a history of hepatitis C. On physical examination, you notice that her vitals are normal. You note well-defined, pruritic, planar, purple, polygonal papules and plaques on her ankles and wrists. Based on her medical history and physical examination, what is the most likely diagnosis?
   a. Leukoplakia
   b. Impetigo
   c. Psoriasis
   d. Lichen planus

159. All of the following are treatments for dyshidrosis EXCEPT:
   a. Antibiotics
   b. Emollients
   c. Steroids
   d. Diphenhydramine

160. A 10-year-old patient has just been diagnosed with diabetes mellitus type 1. What is the first-line medication that you would prescribe?
   a. Metformin
   b. Lantus
   c. Glimepiride
   d. Glyburide

161. A 58-year-old male with a known history of alcohol abuse is brought to the ER for altered mental status. He is oriented to person only, he is vomiting, he is diaphoretic, and you notice a fine tremor. His pupils are dilated, but they are briskly reactive. His vital signs are as follows: BP, 166/89; respirations, 25 per minute; pulse, 119 beats per minute; and pulse oximetry, 95%. He states that he has not had a drink in two days. He denies drug abuse. Based on his medical history and physical examination, what is the most likely diagnosis?
   a. Delusional disorder
   b. Alcohol intoxication
   c. Alcohol withdrawal
   d. Dysthymic disorder

162. A mother brings her 13-year-old son to your office. He has been complaining of persistent unilateral knee pain for several weeks. The pain is exacerbated by movement. The child denies a history of trauma. A prior knee x ray taken in the ER is negative. On physical examination, you notice a painful bony bump just below the affected knee. There is no sign of infection. There is no joint laxity. The child has no medical problems. Based on his medical history and physical examination, what is the most likely diagnosis?
    a. Anterior cruciate ligament (ACL) disruption
    b. Polymyositis
    c. Ganglion cyst
    d. Osgood–Schlatter disease

163. You have a patient that has just been diagnosed with polyarteritis nodosa. What is the next step in your medical management?
    a. Start prednisone
    b. Start clindamycin
    c. Start permethrin
    d. Start amantadine

164. Which of the following is NOT a risk factor for developing condyloma acuminata?
    a. Birth control pills
    b. Late coital age
    c. Smoking
    d. Multiple sex partners

165. An adult patient has an excess of human growth hormone. Which of the following will be the most likely diagnosis?
    a. Gigantism
    b. Dwarfism
    c. Cushing's syndrome
    d. Acromegaly

166. A 35-year-old woman comes to your office with a myriad of complaints. She has noticed fatigue, progressive ataxia, muscle spasms, dizziness, and difficulty with coordination of fine motor movements. She states that she has recently been diagnosed with optic neuritis. What is the most likely diagnosis?
    a. Alzheimer's disease
    b. Meningitis
    c. Multiple sclerosis
    d. Huntington's disease

167. A woman comes to the ER complaining of dry mouth, drooling, right-sided facial swelling, and pain inside of her right cheek. Chewing aggravates the pain. She has had no vocal changes or difficulty with swallowing. Her only medical history is Sjögren's syndrome. What is the most likely diagnosis?
    a. Epiglottitis
    b. Parotitis
    c. Peritonsillar abscess
    d. Oral leukoplakia

168. A five-year-old boy is brought in by his mother to your clinic complaining of sores inside his mouth of three days' duration. She denies fever, discharge from lesions, or trauma. She admits that he's had these lesions before, but they went away on their own. He has no past medical history, and his vitals are normal. On physical examination, you notice two ulcers inside of his lower lip that have a grayish-yellow base and an erythematous halo. What is the next step in your medical management?
    a. Recommend nonsteroidal anti-inflammatory drugs (NSAIDs)
    b. Prescribe oral antiviral medication
    c. Prescribe oral antibiotics
    d. Recommend a decrease in folic acid intake

169. A 13-year-old male patient is brought to the ER with sudden-onset unilateral testicular pain following a trauma that occurred four hours previously. What is the next step in your medical management?
    a. Recommend warm compresses
    b. Stat surgery consult
    c. Order pain medication to see if it alleviates symptoms
    d. Order intravenous (IV) antibiotics

170. A patient is admitted to the ICU with a traumatic head injury. Other than the head injury, the patient has no past medical history. The nurse calls you with the morning labs to let you know that the patient's serum sodium is 150 and the serum potassium is 3.2. The serum glucose and urine glucose are normal. The nurse notes that the patient's urine output has increased to over 300 mL per hour. The urine specific gravity is <1.005. The patient has been drinking profusely throughout the night, but she is still complaining of thirst. Based on the lab results and the patient's medical history, what is the most likely diagnosis?
    a. Hypothyroidism
    b. Diabetes mellitus
    c. Hyperthyroidism
    d. Diabetes insipidus

171. A 35-year-old female comes to your clinic complaining of a painful sore on her neck of several weeks' duration. It keeps changing in appearance. On physical examination, you notice an asymmetric 9 mm papule on the right side of the patient's neck that has mixed areas of brown, blue, and black. It is moderately tender. No discharge can be expressed. There are no other lesions on her body. Based on the patient's medical history and physical examination, what is the most likely diagnosis?
    a. Impetigo
    b. Basal-cell carcinoma
    c. Melanoma
    d. Squamous-cell carcinoma

172. A 61-year-old male comes to the ER with a five-day history of worsening dysuria, hematuria, abdominal pain, and urinary incontinence. He has had an unintentional 15-pound weight loss over the past 30 days. He has a history of smoking one pack of cigarettes per day for 25 years, but he quit smoking five years ago. He has mild tenderness of the bilateral lower quadrants and suprapubic area. Based on his medical history and physical examination, what is the most likely diagnosis?
    a. Wilms' tumor
    b. Prostatitis
    c. Orchitis
    d. Bladder carcinoma

173. A 25-year-old with no past medical history is diagnosed with a corneal abrasion after she tried to remove her contact lens. What is the next step in her medical management?
    a. Gentamicin eyedrops for seven days
    b. Xalatan eyedrops for seven days
    c. Lumigan eyedrops for seven days
    d. Timoptic eyedrops for seven days

174. A patient has just been diagnosed with diabetes insipidus. What is your drug of choice for treating this condition?
    a. Depakote
    b. Decadron
    c. Desmopressin
    d. Detrol

175. A four-year-old child is brought to the ER for the fourth time for first-degree burns. Her right hand and foot have first-degree burns in a "glove and stocking" distribution. The child's prior visits document burns that presented the same way. The mother's explanation is that the child grabbed a hot pan off of the stove. Your next step is to
    a. Call child protective services prior to discharge
    b. Discharge the patient with Silvadene
    c. Discharge the child with Silvadene and po antibiotics
    d. Admit the patient for monitoring

176. Which of the following would NOT be a medical treatment of schizophrenia?
    a. Haldol
    b. Zyprexa
    c. Zofran
    d. Seroquel

177. A patient comes to your office and explains that he has recently been diagnosed with actinic keratosis. What should you advise him to do?
    a. Use antifungal cream
    b. Stay out of the sun
    c. Use steroid cream
    d. Recommend washing all linens in hot water

178. A patient comes to the ER complaining of swelling and pain of the nail bed on her finger for the past several days. The patient states that she had cut her finger several days ago before the symptoms appeared. On physical examination, you notice erythema, tenderness, and swelling of the medial aspect of her nail bed. Scant purulent discharge can be expressed. The patient has no past medical history. What is the most likely diagnosis?
    a. Scabies
    b. Paronychia
    c. Onychomycosis
    d. Condyloma acuminata

179. A patient comes to your clinic with widespread symmetrical loss of pigmentation of his or her skin. What is the most likely diagnosis?
    a. Lipoma
    b. Xanthelasma
    c. Mongolian spots
    d. Vitiligo

180. Which of the following medications would NOT be recommended in a patient with a history of fecal impaction?
    a. Colace
    b. Senna
    c. Morphine
    d. Milk of Magnesia

181. Which of the following medications may be administered to a patient who is having an episode of supraventricular tachycardia?
    a. Atropine
    b. Allopurinol
    c. Atorvastatin
    d. Adenosine

182. A patient presents with shortness of breath, dizziness, and chest pain. An electrocardiogram (EKG) shows sinus bradycardia. The patient's vital signs are as follows: BP, 101/55; pulse, 31 beats per minute; respirations, 18 per minute; and oxygen saturation, 96% on room air. What is the next step in your medical management?
    a. Give atropine
    b. Give amiodarone
    c. Give vasopressin
    d. Give adenosine

183. A patient in your office had blood drawn as part of her annual visit. On her blood work, you notice her HBsAg is negative, her anti-HBc is negative, and her anti-HBs is positive. Based on her lab values, what is the diagnosis?
    a. She is susceptible to being infected with hepatitis B
    b. She is chronically infected with hepatitis B
    c. She is immune due to hepatitis B due to prior vaccination
    d. She is acutely infected with hepatitis B

184. You are seeing a patient with suspected giant-cell arteritis. What is the next step in your management?
    a. Start on po antibiotics
    b. Recommend oncology referral for chemotherapy
    c. Monitor for now
    d. Recommend vascular surgery referral for biopsy

185. A patient in your office had blood drawn as part of her annual visit. You notice that her thyroid-stimulating hormone (TSH) level is high, her T3 level is normal, and her T4 level is low. Based on her lab values, what is the diagnosis?
    a. Addison's disease
    b. Hypothyroidism
    c. Hyperthyroidism
    d. Graves' disease

186. Which of the following medications may be useful in shortening the course of influenza if given early enough in the course of infection?
    a. Oseltamivir
    b. Acyclovir
    c. Famciclovir
    d. Augmentin

187. A patient is ambulating with physical therapy in the ICU when one of the therapists tells you that the patient's blood pressure went from 155/88 in the supine position to 131/70 in the sitting position. The other vital signs are as follows: pulse, 99; respirations, 18 per minute; and oxygen saturation, 97% on room air. The patient is now complaining of dizziness and headache. The patient's electrocardiogram (EKG) is normal. What is the most likely diagnosis?
    a. Sick sinus syndrome
    b. Angina
    c. Orthostatic hypotension
    d. Atrial fibrillation

188. A 68-year-old male presents to the ER with headache and nausea. A computed tomography (CT) scan of his head, electrocardiogram (EKG), and troponin level are normal. The urinalysis shows proteinuria. The patient's vital signs are as follows: pulse, 98 beats per minute; respirations, 16 per minute; and BP, 205/121. What is the most likely diagnosis?
    a. Stage 2 hypertension
    b. Hypertensive crisis
    c. Prehypertension
    d. Stage 1 hypertension

189. A 27-year-old obese female comes to your clinic complaining of worsening fatigue and frequent urination of several weeks' duration. Her urinalysis is positive for glucose and yeast. Her vital signs are normal. What is the next step in your medical management?
    a. Order ciprofloxacin and Pyridium
    b. Order a urine culture and blood cultures
    c. Order a repeat urinalysis in two weeks
    d. Order a hemoglobin A1C (HA1C) test, complete blood count (CBC), and basic metabolic panel (BMP)

190. A 21-year-old male comes to the ER with worsening left-sided testicular pain and swelling of three days' duration. He denies trauma. He has no past medical history. His vitals are normal. On physical examination, you palpate his scrotum, which feels like there's a mass of worms inside. Based on his medical history and physical, the most likely diagnosis is
    a. Hydrocele
    b. Varicocele
    c. Testicular torsion
    d. Testicular carcinoma

191. A patient comes to your clinic complaining of worsening diaphoresis, palpitations, and generalized tremor for several weeks. On physical examination, you notice that the patient has exophthalmos. What is the most likely diagnosis?
   a. Graves' disease
   b. Addison's disease
   c. Cushing's disease
   d. Hashimoto's disease

192. A 24-year-old male comes to the ER complaining of fever, chills, groin pain, dysuria, painful ejaculation, and testicular swelling of two days' duration. He denies trauma. What is the most likely diagnosis?
   a. Pyelonephritis
   b. Epididymitis
   c. Prostatitis
   d. Cystitis

193. A patient comes to your clinic for his annual purified protein derivative (PPD) injection. The patient works as a nurse at a local hospital. What is the minimum diameter of induration for a positive PPD test in this patient?
   a. 2 mm
   b. 5 mm
   c. 10 mm
   d. 15 mm

194. You have just examined a patient and suspect that she has Graves' disease. What is the next step in your medical management?
   a. Order thyroid function tests
   b. Order a complete endocrine panel
   c. Order a cortisol level
   d. Order a hemoglobin A1C (HA1C)

195. A woman with a history of bipolar disorder presents to the ER with altered mental status. She was intubated by emergency medical services (EMS) when she was found to be unconscious by the team. Her family notes that she was on lithium for her bipolar disorder. Her lithium level is high. Her blood urea nitrogen (BUN) and creatinine are 96/3.2. The patient is anuric. What is the immediate next course of medical action?
   a. Dialysis
   b. Fluid hydration
   c. Repeat lithium level in 12 hours
   d. Repeat BUN/creatinine in 12 hours

196. Which of the following groups is NOT recommended to get the flu vaccine?
   a. Adults age 50 and older
   b. Pregnant women
   c. Children less than 6 months old
   d. Health-care workers

197. A 44-year-old female presents to the ER with worsening nausea, vomiting, and diarrhea. She notes that she's been craving salty foods recently. Her vital signs are as follows: BP, 88/55; pulse, 66 beats per minute; respirations, 14 per minute; pulse oximetry, 98% on room air; and temperature, 98.9 °F. You notice that her skin has patchy areas of hyperpigmentation, which appear as if she had gone tanning. What is the most likely diagnosis?
  a. Hashimoto's disease
  b. Graves' disease
  c. Cushing's disease
  d. Addison's disease

198. A patient comes to your office complaining of headache, persistent urinary tract infections, unintentional weight loss, and fatigue. His fasting serum glucose is 161. His hemoglobin A1C (HA1C) is 6.2. His vitals are normal. His body mass index (BMI) is normal. He has no past medical problems. What is your medical recommendation to this patient?
  a. Lose weight
  b. Modify diet
  c. Start metformin
  d. Start insulin

199. A patient comes to your office complaining of erectile dysfunction. Which of the following medications would you NOT prescribe for this condition?
  a. Cialis
  b. Levitra
  c. Viagra
  d. Propecia

200. A patient with no past medical history had a purified protein derivative (PPD) shot three days ago and now has an induration of 5 mm. She works as a librarian. What is the next step in your medical management?
  a. Order a chest x ray
  b. Order a repeat PPD in one month
  c. No intervention for now
  d. Start tuberculosis medications

201. A 24-year-old male comes to your clinic complaining of having epididymitis. He states that he's had several prior epididymitis infections. He notes that he is sexually active and occasionally does not use protection. He denies other medical problems. What would you advise this patient?
  a. Increase fluid intake
  b. Avoid red meat, seafood, and alcohol
  c. Use protection when having intercourse
  d. Recommend urology referral

202. During a colonoscopy, it is discovered that a patient has multiple areas of outpouching along the colonic wall. What is the most likely diagnosis?
  a. Intussusception
  b. Diverticulosis
  c. Mallory–Weiss tear
  d. Celiac sprue

203. You suspect that a patient has septic arthritis. Which of the following would NOT be part of your medical management?
a. Prescribe colchicine
b. Perform a joint aspiration
c. Order blood cultures
d. Prescribe nonsteroidal anti-inflammatory drugs (NSAIDs)

204. You have just diagnosed a patient with celiac disease. What is the next step in your medical management?
a. Prescribe antibiotics
b. Order blood cultures
c. Surgery referral
d. Recommend dietary modifications

205. A 40-year-old male patient comes to the ER complaining of left-lower extremity pain. He is diagnosed with a blood clot in his left soleal vein. He has a past medical history of hypertension and hyperlipidemia. What is the next step in your medical management?
a. Discharge home and get follow up Doppler ultrasound in two weeks
b. Start Coumadin as an outpatient
c. Admit the patient and start a Heparin infusion and Coumadin
d. Surgery consult for placement of an inferior vena cava (IVC) filter

206. A mother brings her three-year-old son to the ER, stating that he fell on the playground earlier and then he stopped using his left arm. On physical examination, the child is holding his left arm flexed and pronated. He is not in any pain or distress as long as his arm is maintained in that position. There is no swelling, deformity, or discoloration of the extremity. Based on his medical history and physical examination, what is the most likely diagnosis?
a. Lisfranc fracture
b. Colles' fracture
c. Nursemaid's elbow
d. Greenstick fracture

207. A one-month-old baby girl born full term is diagnosed with patent ductus arteriosus (PDA). Her vital signs and physical examination are normal. What is the next step in your medical management?
a. Recommend cardiology evaluation for possible surgical closure
b. No intervention for now
c. Prescribe aspirin 81 mg
d. Prescribe indomethacin

208. A patient has just been diagnosed with benign prostatic hypertrophy. Which of the following medication would you NOT prescribe for this condition?
a. Proscar
b. Cardura
c. Rapaflo
d. Ramipril

209. You are seeing a 58-year-old patient in the ER who you think may be having an acute cerebral vascular accident. His symptoms started 30 minutes ago. His past medical history includes hypertension, obesity, and hyperlipidemia. His vital signs are normal. What is the next step in your medical management?
    a. Start a heparin infusion
    b. Reassess his examination in 30 minutes
    c. Administer tissue plasminogen activator (tPA)
    d. Order a computed tomography (CT) scan of the brain

210. A patient is diagnosed with *Clostridium difficile* colitis. The patient has no allergies to medication. Which of the following medications would you prescribe?
    a. Vancomycin po
    b. Clindamycin po
    c. IV azithromycin
    d. IV vancomycin

211. Which of the following medications would help treat a patient in status epilepticus?
    a. Levetiracetam and linezolid
    b. Phenylephrine and Lomotil
    c. Phenytoin and lorazepam
    d. Phenytoin and linezolid

212. Which medical triad includes three factors thought to contribute to thrombosis?
    a. Beck's triad
    b. Virchow's triad
    c. Charcot's triad
    d. Cushing's triad

213. A patient comes to the ER with right-sided foot pain after accidentally striking his foot against a baseboard. He has moderate pain at the first and second metatarsals with mild swelling with palpable deformity. Based on his medical history and physical, what is the most likely diagnosis?
    a. Le Fort fracture
    b. Lisfranc fracture
    c. Monteggia fracture
    d. Colles' fracture

214. A patient with cystic fibrosis asks you what medications she can take to help decrease her risk of secondary infection. Which of the following medications would you NOT advise this patient to take?
    a. Motrin
    b. Amiodarone
    c. Mucinex
    d. Albuterol

215. Which of the following is a complication of pulmonary tuberculosis?
    a. Parkinson's disease
    b. Hashimoto's disease
    c. Cushing's disease
    d. Pott's disease

216. A patient comes to your clinic complaining of pains all over her body. Multiple lab tests and scans have been negative for acute pathology. She has a history of depression. What is the most likely diagnosis?
  a. Fibromyalgia
  b. Polyarteritis nodosa
  c. Osteoarthritis
  d. Polymyalgia rheumatica

217. Which of the following medications would be used for a person diagnosed with generalized anxiety disorder?
  a. Prednisolone
  b. Promethazine
  c. Permethrin
  d. Paroxetine

218. A 68-year-old woman comes to your clinic complaining of decreasing vision in her left eye for the past several weeks. She noticed that she has problems differentiating between contrasts and identifying colors. She denies headache, trauma, and eye pain or discharge from the eye. She has no significant past medical history. She has a clouding of her left lens. What is the most likely diagnosis?
  a. Hyphema
  b. Blepharitis
  c. Cataract
  d. Conjunctivitis

219. You suspect a patient has a deep venous thrombus. Which of the following tests should you initially order?
  a. X ray
  b. Doppler ultrasound
  c. Computed tomography (CT) scan
  d. Magnetic resonance imaging (MRI)

220. A bleeding defect is seen in the distal esophagus of a patient during an esophagogastroduodenoscopy. The patient has a known history of alcoholism. What is the most likely diagnosis?
  a. Mallory–Weiss tear
  b. Crohn's disease
  c. Ulcerative colitis
  d. Whipple's disease

221. A 66-year-old female comes to the ER complaining of right calf pain and swelling of 12 hours' duration. She has a past medical history of arthritis and osteoporosis. She states that she had a right hip replacement four days ago. On physical examination, you note that she has a positive Homan's sign. Based on her medical history and physical examination, what is the most likely diagnosis?
  a. Septic arthritis
  b. Osgood–Schlatter disease
  c. Osteomyelitis
  d. Venous thrombus

222. While reviewing a two-dimensional echocardiography (2D echo) with a cardiologist, you both see that there is backflow of blood from the left ventricle into the left atrium. What is this condition called?
   a. Mitral regurgitation
   b. Pulmonic regurgitation
   c. Tricuspid regurgitation
   d. Aortic regurgitation

223. A patient in the intensive care unit (ICU) suddenly goes into pulseless ventricular tachycardia. What is one of the first medications you would administer?
   a. Magnesium sulfate
   b. Lidocaine
   c. Epinephrine
   d. Amiodarone

224. Parents bring their 13-year-old son into your clinic for his annual physical evaluation. They have expressed concern because they have noticed that the child has been developing breasts over the past year, which has been a source of anxiety and distress for their son. On physical examination, you notice that the child has enlarged mammary glands bilaterally. The child has no past medical history. The rest of his physical examination is normal. Based on the medical history and physical examination, what is the most likely diagnosis?
   a. Fibrocystic breast disease
   b. Gynecomastia
   c. Fibroadenoma
   d. Carcinoma

225. Parents bring in their two-year-old child to your clinic. They note that he has been tugging on his ears for the past two days. He has been getting over a viral upper respiratory infection, but he is otherwise healthy. Upon physical examination, you notice that his left tympanic membrane is erythematous and bulging. His physical examination is otherwise normal. Based on the medical history and physical examination, what is the most likely diagnosis?
   a. Otitis media
   b. Mastoiditis
   c. Otitis externa
   d. Acoustic neuroma

226. A 45-year-old male with a known history of human immunodeficiency virus (HIV) is brought to the ER with sudden onset of confusion, nausea, vomiting, neck pain, headache, and photophobia. There is no history of trauma. A computed tomography (CT) scan without contrast of the head and neck is negative for acute pathology. Upon physical examination, you note that the patient has a positive Kerning's sign. Based on the medical history and physical examination, what is the most likely diagnosis?
   a. Guillain–Barré syndrome
   b. Meningitis
   c. Huntington's disease
   d. Schistosomiasis

227. A patient with an unknown infection undergoes a lumbar puncture. The lumbar puncture results show an elevated opening pressure, elevated white blood cell count, elevated neutrophil count, and decreased glucose level. Based on the results, what is the most likely diagnosis?
    a. Huntington's disease
    b. Bacterial meningitis
    c. Viral meningitis
    d. Myasthenia gravis

228. A blood gas shows the following results: pH, 7.31; $PaCO_2$, 50; $HCO_3$, 25; and $PaO_2$, 94. Which of the following is the most likely diagnosis?
    a. Metabolic alkalosis
    b. Respiratory alkalosis
    c. Metabolic acidosis
    d. Respiratory acidosis

229. A 26-year-old patient is brought to the ER by his family for sudden onset of dementia, ataxia, and urinary incontinence of four days' duration. He has recently recovered from a cerebral aneurysm rupture. A computed tomography (CT) scan shows distended ventricles. A lumbar puncture is performed, but the results are normal. What is the most likely diagnosis?
    a. Medulloblastoma
    b. Intraventricular hemorrhage
    c. Normal pressure hydrocephalus (NPH)
    d. Hygroma

230. A 15-year-old female is brought to your clinic by her mother, who states that her child has not been eating. The girl has no past medical history. Upon further discussion, the child confides in you that she purposely has been skipping meals so she can lose weight. What is the most likely diagnosis?
    a. Anorexia nervosa
    b. Bulimia nervosa
    c. Generalized anxiety disorder
    d. Bipolar disorder

231. A 40-year-old male comes to your clinic and reports that he feels nervous all of the time. He has no history of personal loss, disturbing life event, or illness. His physical examination and vital signs are normal. He has no medical problems. What is the most likely diagnosis?
    a. Dysthymic disorder
    b. Generalized anxiety disorder
    c. Posttraumatic stress disorder
    d. Phobia

232. A patient in the intensive care unit has the following blood gas: pH, 7.47; $PaCO_2$, 39; $HCO_3$, 29. What is the most likely diagnosis?
    a. Respiratory acidosis
    b. Respiratory alkalosis
    c. Metabolic alkalosis
    d. Metabolic acidosis

233. A patient with normal pressure hydrocephalus undergoes a lumbar puncture. The patient's symptoms improve. What is the next step in this patient's management?
   a. Obtain a magnetic resonance imaging (MRI) scan of the brain
   b. Repeat the lumbar puncture in 48 hours
   c. Ventricular peritoneal shunt
   d. Perform an electroencephalogram (EEG)

234. A patient comes to your clinic for an annual physical examination. The patient confesses to you that she has a hard time coming to your clinic, or being outside in general, because of her fear of being outdoors. She reports feelings of extreme anxiety once she leaves her house. She denies any reason for her to be nervous of crowds of people. What is the most likely diagnosis?
   a. Generalized anxiety disorder
   b. Posttraumatic stress disorder
   c. Dysthymic disorder
   d. Phobia disorder

235. A patient has hypertrophic cardiomyopathy. What is the most common cause for this condition?
   a. Genetic mutation
   b. Disease
   c. Infection
   d. Cancer

236. Parents bring their child into the ER stating that the child has developed rapid, uncontrolled body movements and a fever of 102° F at home. You notice these body movements during your physical examination as well. You draw blood for lab work, which shows that the patient has a white blood cell count of 17,000 as well as an elevated erythrocyte sedimentation rate (ESR). Which of the following signs/symptoms is not part of the minor manifestations of rheumatic fever according to the Jones criteria?
   a. Fever
   b. Chorea
   c. Leukocytosis
   d. Elevated ESR

237. You are reviewing a two-dimensional echocardiogram when you notice backflow of blood from the right ventricle into the right atrium. The most likely diagnosis is
   a. Aortic regurgitation
   b Mitral regurgitation
   c. Pulmonic regurgitation
   d. Tricuspid regurgitation

238. Which of the following medications should NOT be given in a patient with pulseless ventricular fibrillation?
   a. Amiodarone
   b. Lidocaine
   c. Vasopressin
   d. Atropine

239. A nurse hands you the following arterial blood gas results: pH, 7.49; $PaCO_2$, 20; and $HCO_3$, 23. Which of the following is the most likely diagnosis?
a. Metabolic alkalosis
b. Respiratory alkalosis
c. Metabolic acidosis
d. Respiratory acidosis

240. A patient is brought to the ER for acute alcohol intoxication. As the patient begins to wake up, you notice persistent, involuntary, horizontal eye movements of both eyes. What is the most likely diagnosis?
a. Conjunctivitis
b. Nystagmus
c. Entropion
d. Exotropia

241. A patient arrives in the ER complaining of chest pain, dizziness, and shortness of breath. An electrocardiogram (EKG) shows a secondary R wave in lead V1 and a widened QRS complex. What is this conduction disorder called?
a. Torsades de pointes
b. Right bundle branch block
c. Atrial fibrillation
d. Sinus tachycardia

242. A 65-year-old male patient presents to the ER with dysarthria, ataxia, and left-sided weakness, which occurred for about 30 minutes and then spontaneously resolved. His physical examination is normal. A computed tomography (CT) scan of the brain is normal. What is the most likely diagnosis?
a. Transient ischemic attack
b. Cerebral aneurysm rupture
c. Cerebral vascular accident
d. Migraine

243. A patient with a known history of anxiety and depression is in your clinic for a routine physical examination and confides in you that he wants to commit suicide. He tells you how and when he plans to do it. Which of the following is NOT an appropriate action as a medical professional?
a. Advise the patient to call a suicide hotline
b. Obtain a stat psychiatric referral
c. Do not report the patient's actions
d. Advise the patient's spouse or parents of his intent

244. A patient comes to your clinic complaining of persistent right-eye irritation. The conjunctiva is normal. You note that the patient's right lower lid is turned inward. What is this condition called?
a. Entropion
b. Exotropia
c. Ectropion
d. Esotropia

245. Parents bring in their five-year-old son for his annual physical examination. The parents state that their son has been having trouble at school and at home for frequent temper tantrums, angry outbursts, short temper, and hostility toward others. He hasn't gone through any life-threatening situations, suffered personal losses, or had any recent changes in his life. His physical examination and vital signs are normal. He has no past medical history. What is the most likely diagnosis?
    a. Adjustment disorder
    b. Dysthymic disorder
    c. Attention-deficit hyperactivity disorder
    d. Oppositional-defiant disorder

246. One of your patients has been diagnosed with phlebitis. Which of the following would NOT be a part of your medical management?
    a. Prescribe Colchicine
    b. Recommend compression stockings
    c. Prescribe analgesics
    d. Recommend warm compresses

247. A patient comes to the ER with palpitations, chest pain, dizziness, and shortness of breath. An electrocardiogram (EKG) shows a heart rate of 120 beats per minute. The EKG shows irregular QRS complexes and no P waves. What is the most likely diagnosis?
    a. Right bundle branch block
    b. Sinus tachycardia
    c. Atrial fibrillation
    d. Sinus bradycardia

248. A 16-year-old female patient arrives in the ER complaining of headache, nausea, and photophobia. She is diagnosed with a migraine headache. Which of the following medications would you prescribe for this patient to help prevent and treat future episodes?
    a. Fluvastatin
    b. Frovatriptan
    c. Fluoxetine
    d. Fexofenadine

249. A patient is diagnosed with Guillain–Barré syndrome. Which of the following is NOT a method to reduce symptoms, prevent complications, and speed up recovery?
    a. Plasmapheresis
    b. Intubation
    c. Immunoglobulin therapy
    d. Lumbar puncture

250. A 21-year-old male patient arrives in your office for the first time for a routine physical examination. While talking to him, you note that he has involuntary facial tics. His cognitive function is normal. What is the most likely diagnosis for his behavior?
    a. Huntington's disease
    b. Tourette disorder
    c. Alzheimer's disease
    d. Multiple sclerosis

251. You are examining a patient with suspected chronic obstructive pulmonary disease (COPD). Which of the following is the best test to help aid your diagnosis?
a. Spirometry
b. Chest x ray
c. Auscultation with a stethoscope
d. Electrocardiogram (EKG)

252. Which of the following tests is the most sensitive for detecting cystic fibrosis?
a. Chest x ray
b. Fecal fat test
c. Sweat chloride test
d. Computed tomography (CT) scan of the chest

253. A patient arrives in the ER complaining of worsening hemoptysis, fever, chills, and weakness for the past week. This patient has a history of human immunodeficiency virus (HIV). A chest x ray is ordered, which shows a fungal ball in the right lung. What is the most likely diagnosis?
a. Cystic fibrosis
b. Pneumoconiosis
c. Sarcoidosis
d. Aspergillosis

254. A mother brings in her 18-month-old son to your clinic, noting that he has been displaying progressively deteriorating social and communication skills and repetitive behaviors. This triad of symptoms best defines which of the following disorders?
a. Oppositional-defiant disorder
b. Attention-deficit hyperactivity disorder
c. Autism disorder
d. Adjustment disorder

255. A mother pregnant with her first child is Rh-positive. The child is Rh-positive. What is the next step in medical management?
a. Prescribe antibiotics
b. Order an ultrasound
c. No intervention
d. Prescribe RhoGAM

256. A woman who is 36 weeks pregnant develops eclampsia. Her liver function tests and complete blood count are normal. What would be the next step in medical management?
a. Observe on telemetry monitor
b. Discharge home and monitor as an outpatient
c. Induce labor
d. Order a stat blood transfusion

257. A 56-year-old man with a history of chronic obstructive pulmonary disease (COPD) comes to the ER complaining of worsening shortness of breath and chest pain. A chest x ray shows blunting of the right costophrenic angle. What is the most likely diagnosis?
a. Pleural effusion
b. Aspergillosis
c. Pneumoconiosis
d. Pneumothorax

258. Which of the following chest x-ray findings is most consistent with the diagnosis of a pneumothorax whose size is approximately 5%?
   a. Honeycomb appearance of the lungs
   b. Granulomas
   c. Area on chest x ray with no lung markings
   d. Normal chest x ray

259. Which of the following conditions would NOT be a contributing factor to the development of obesity?
   a. Graves' disease
   b. Hypothyroidism
   c. Cushing's syndrome
   d. Menopause

260. Which of the following is NOT a treatment for allergic rhinitis?
   a. Decongestants
   b. Antihistamines
   c. Antibiotics
   d. Corticosteroids

261. Which of the following would NOT be used in the treatment of a patient with a phobia disorder?
   a. Xanax
   b. Metoprolol
   c. Lexapro
   d. Ritalin

262. Which of the following treatments is NOT an intervention for a patient going through withdrawal from alcohol?
   a. Zofran
   b. Narcan
   c. Thiamine
   d. Ativan

263. A 37-year-old female patient comes to the ER complaining of worsening fever, dysphonia, and dysphagia of three days' duration. She notes recently having a tooth infection, but she did not seek medical attention for it. While you are talking to the patient, her family member says, "she sounds like she has a hot potato in her mouth." Her tongue is swollen and out of place, and she has swelling and erythema of her proximal neck. What is the most likely diagnosis?
   a. Oral leukoplakia
   b. Acute pharyngitis
   c. Ludwig's angina
   d. Aphthous ulcers

264. A patient being seen in the ER is diagnosed with a blowout fracture. Which of the following would NOT be an intervention for this patient?
   a. Irrigation
   b. Antibiotics
   c. Steroids
   d. Surgery

265. A patient comes to the ER complaining of facial pain and swelling after being physically assaulted. A computed tomography (CT) scan reveals a fractured maxilla. What is the most likely diagnosis?
   a. Boxer's fracture
   b. Lisfranc fracture
   c. Colles' fracture
   d. Le Fort fracture

266. What is the most common preventable cause of pelvic inflammatory disease?
   a. Appendicitis
   b. Ectopic pregnancy
   c. Childbirth
   d. Venereal disease

267. A patient is diagnosed with gastroesophageal reflux disease. Which of the following medications is the most appropriate treatment for this condition?
   a. Ketoconazole
   b. Metronidazole
   c. Fluconazole
   d. Esomeprazole

268. Which of the following statements is FALSE regarding Meckel's diverticulum?
   a. It is more common in females than males
   b. It is usually found about two feet from the ileocecal valve
   c. Initial presentation is more common in toddlers than adults
   d. It affects approximately 2% of the population

269. A patient comes to your clinic complaining of worsening gastroesophageal reflux symptoms as well as abdominal pain and hematemesis. A serum gastrin level is high. A computed tomography (CT) scan of the abdomen shows multiple small tumors in the head of the pancreas and the duodenum. What is the most likely diagnosis?
   a. Celiac disease
   b. Zollinger–Ellison syndrome
   c. Whipple's disease
   d. Crohn's disease

270. A patient comes to the ER with increasing left shoulder pain and decreased range of motion after a heavy box fell on his shoulder. On physical examination, he has limited abduction. A shoulder x ray is negative for fracture or dislocation. What is the next step in your medical management?
   a. Order a repeat x ray in two weeks
   b. Order a magnetic resonance imaging (MRI) scan of the shoulder
   c. No intervention
   d. Administer electromyography (EMG)

271. A patient is admitted to the hospital for multiple right leg fractures following a motor vehicle accident. The leg is casted, and the patient is sent to the intensive care unit (ICU) for monitoring. A nurse calls you later on that day to tell you that the patient's right foot has become pale and cold. An arterial ultrasound shows no flow. His creatine phosphokinase (CPK) level is 14,000. What is the most likely diagnosis?
   a. Osgood–Schlatter disease
   b. Deep venous thrombosis
   c. Compartment syndrome
   d. Septic arthritis

272. A patient is diagnosed with trichomoniasis. What is the next step in your medical management?
   a. Rocephin
   b. Metronidazole
   c. Azithromycin
   d. Fluconazole

273. A patient comes to your clinic stating that she has noticed skin changes over her right breast. During the physical examination, you note that her skin has a swollen, pitted surface. What is the most likely diagnosis?
   a. Carcinoma
   b. Abscess
   c. Gynecomastia
   d. Fibroadenoma

274. Which of the following will not help alleviate the symptoms of premenstrual syndrome?
   a. Exercise
   b. Dietary modifications
   c. Birth control pills
   d. Caffeine

275. Which of the following will NOT help prevent cervical cancer?
   a. Regular Pap smears
   b. Limit tobacco abuse
   c. Cease having children
   d. Limit the number of sexual partners

276. Which of the following is the best way to prevent beriberi?
   a. Increase calcium intake
   b. Increase thiamine intake
   c. Increase folate intake
   d. Increase iron intake

277. Which of the following is the best way to prevent osteoporosis?
   a. Increase calcium intake
   b. Increase thiamine intake
   c. Increase folate intake
   d. Increase iron intake

278. A friend is telling you about a family member who suffers from a disease resulting is misshapen bones and persistent pathologic fractures. The most likely diagnosis for this condition is
   a. Septic arthritis
   b. Paget's disease
   c. Osteosarcoma
   d. Wilms' tumor

279. A woman who is 35 weeks pregnant presents to the ER with continuous contractions, abdominal pain, back pain, and bright-red vaginal bleeding. What is the most likely diagnosis?
   a. Endometriosis
   b. Premature rupture of the membranes
   c. Placental abruption (abruptio placentae)
   d. Placenta previa

280. A 23-year-old male complaining of right knee pain after a football injury two days ago comes to the ER. His right knee is diffusely swollen, and he has difficulty putting weight on his right leg. The patient has a positive Lachman test. What is the most likely diagnosis?
   a. Posterior cruciate ligament tear
   b. Lateral collateral ligament tear
   c. Medial collateral ligament tear
   d. Anterior cruciate ligament tear

281. A patient comes to the ER complaining of left wrist pain after falling on an outstretched hand. An x ray shows a fracture of the distal radius and a dislocation at the radioulnar joint. What is the most likely diagnosis?
   a. Le Fort fracture
   b. Colles' fracture
   c. Galeazzi fracture
   d. Monteggia fracture

282. An x ray shows a transverse and mildly displaced fourth metacarpal fracture. The patient had come to the ER complaining of hand pain after being involved in a physical altercation. What is the most likely diagnosis?
   a. Colles' fracture
   b. Lisfranc fracture
   c. Hangman's fracture
   d. Boxer's fracture

283. A 24-year-old female who is 12 weeks pregnant comes to the ER complaining of sudden-onset abdominal pain and vaginal bleeding. She has had a prior transvaginal ultrasound, which showed an intrauterine pregnancy (IUP). An ultrasound cannot visualize the IUP. A urine pregnancy test is negative. What is the most likely diagnosis?
   a. Threatened abortion
   b. Missed abortion
   c. Completed abortion
   d Dysmenorrhea

284. A patient comes to the ER with nausea, vomiting, and constipation for two days. The patient was discharged from the hospital a week before after having a laparoscopic appendectomy. An abdominal x ray shows a distended bowel without evidence of obstruction. What is the most likely diagnosis?
   a. Gastroesophageal reflux disease
   b. Ileus
   c. Toxic megacolon
   d. Irritable bowel syndrome

285. Which of the following would NOT be an appropriate treatment for giardiasis?
   a. Furosemide
   b. Ondansetron
   c. Loperamide
   d. Metronidazole

286. Which of the following tests is NOT appropriate in the workup of lactose intolerance?
   a. Lactose tolerance test
   b. Lactose-hydrogen breath test
   c. Serum calcium
   d. Stool pH

287. Which of the following tests is the most diagnostic for monitoring the course of choriocarcinoma and its response to therapy?
   a. Complete blood cell count
   b. Bence Jones protein
   c. Computed tomography (CT) scan of the abdomen and pelvis
   d. Beta human chorionic gonadotropin (hCG)

288. All of the following are therapies used to treat leiomyomas EXCEPT
   a. Nonsteroidal anti-inflammatory drugs (NSAIDs)
   b. Birth control pills
   c. Antibiotics
   d. Iron supplements

289. A 16-year-old female comes to the office with worsening pelvic pain, dysmenorrhea, throbbing pain that radiates down her legs, and dysuria for several weeks. She is not sexually active. She has no past medical history. Abdominal and pelvic ultrasounds are negative. A urine pregnancy test is negative. She undergoes a laparoscopy, which shows multiple dark-colored lesions on the ovaries, outside of the uterus, and on the abdominal wall. What is the most likely diagnosis?
   a. Dystocia
   b. Leiomyoma
   c. Choriocarcinoma
   d. Endometriosis

290. Which of the following would NOT be a treatment for sciatica?
   a. Nonsteroidal anti-inflammatory drugs (NSAIDs)
   b. Corticosteroid injections
   c. Surgery
   d. Physical therapy

291. A 17-year-old female is brought to your clinic for worsening pain and swelling of her knees, elbows, and hips. She has recently developed a butterfly-shaped rash that covers the bridge of her nose and her cheeks. There is no history of trauma. She has no significant past medical history. X rays of the knees, elbows, and hips are normal. What is the most likely diagnosis?
    a. Systemic lupus erythematous
    b. Paget's disease
    c. Polymyositis
    d. Huntington's disease

292. Which of the following is NOT an appropriate intervention for a partial small-bowel obstruction?
    a. Antibiotics
    b. Intravenous (IV) fluids
    c. Nasogastric tube
    d. Antiemetic medications

293. A patient comes to your office complaining of alternating episodes of diarrhea and constipation that get worse after eating. Her lab tests are normal, her colonoscopy is normal, and a computed tomography (CT) scan of the abdomen and pelvis is normal. The symptoms are not caused by one particular type of food. She has a known history of anxiety and depression. What is the most likely diagnosis?
    a. Irritable bowel syndrome
    b. Crohn's disease
    c. Ulcerative colitis
    d. Toxic megacolon

294. A patient is diagnosed with pelvic inflammatory disease. Which of the following is the most appropriate treatment for this condition?
    a. Antifungal medications
    b. Antibiotics
    c. Antiviral medications
    d. No treatment is necessary

295. A patient is diagnosed with polymyositis. Which of the following is the most appropriate treatment for this condition?
    a. Antibiotics
    b. Nonsteroidal anti-inflammatory drugs (NSAIDs)
    c. Antiviral medications
    d. Corticosteroids

296. What is the primary underlying cause of spondylolisthesis?
    a. Incorrect alignment of the disc
    b. Insufficient calcium
    c. Unknown cause
    d. Infectious etiology

297. Which of the following is the least effective method of preventing unwanted pregnancy?
    a. Intrauterine device
    b. Birth control pills
    c. Withdrawal method
    d. Condoms

298. Which of the following medications is the most appropriate in treating rheumatoid arthritis?
   a. Metronidazole
   b. Meropenem
   c. Metformin
   d. Methotrexate

299. Which of the following is a major contributing factor to the development of osteoarthritis?
   a. Immune disorder
   b. Degenerative disease
   c. Congenital disorder
   d. Infectious etiology

300. An 82-year-old male with a known history of osteoarthritis comes to your clinic complaining of worsening back pain. During the examination, you notice he has a C-shaped curvature of his spine, causing him to look like a hunchback. What is the most likely diagnosis for this condition?
   a. Kyphosis
   b. Cauda equina syndrome
   c. Avascular necrosis
   d. Sciatica

# Answers and Explanations

1. C: Cushing's triad is a clinical triad defined as hypertension, bradycardia, and irregular respirations. It suggests rising intracranial pressure due to intracranial pathology such as hemorrhage.
Beck's triad is the combination of distended jugular veins, hypotension, and muffled heart sounds. It occurs as a result of pericardial effusion.
Charcot's triad is the combination of jaundice, fever, and right-upper quadrant abdominal pain. It occurs as a result of ascending cholangitis.
Bergman's triad is the combination of dyspnea, petechiae, and mental status changes. It occurs when a patient has a fat embolism.

2. A: **Major manifestations of acute rheumatic fever include the following:**
Erythema marginatum: raised, nonpruritic, pink rings on the trunk and inner surfaces of the limbs
Carditis: inflammation of the heart muscle
Chorea: rapid, uncontrolled body movements
Subcutaneous nodules: painless, firm collections of collagen fibers over bones or tendons
Polyarthritis: temporary migrating inflammation of the large joints

**Minor manifestations of acute rheumatic fever include the following:**
1) Fever (101 °F to 102 °F)
2) Arthralgia: joint pain without swelling
3) Elevated erythrocyte sedimentation rate (ESR) or C-reactive protein (CRP)
4) Leukocytosis
5) Prior episode of rheumatic heart disease
6) Heart block seen on an electrocardiogram (EKG)

3. D: Psoriasis causes cells to build up rapidly on the surface of the skin, forming itchy, dry, red, raised patches covered with grayish silvery lesions that are easily friable. Psoriasis is sometimes painful. Plaques frequently occur on the skin of the elbows and knees, but they can affect any area. This is a chronic condition.
Impetigo is a bacterial infection that is most commonly caused by *Staphylococcus aureus* or *Streptococcus pyogenes*. It causes lesions that can occur anywhere on the body. They are small, red, and pus-filled and can crack open and form a yellow or honey-colored, thick crust. They occur most commonly in young children.
Tinea corporis, also known as "ringworm," is a fungal infection that develops on the superficial layer of the skin, occurring anywhere on the body. It is characterized by an itchy, red, circular rash with a central clearing.
Rosacea is a chronic inflammatory skin condition characterized by redness of the face, most commonly on the cheeks, nose, and forehead.

4. B: In Crohn's disease, the colon wall may have a "cobblestone" appearance due to the intermittent pattern of affected and nonaffected colonic tissue.
Celiac sprue is an immune reaction that damages the lining of the small intestine and prevents it from absorbing important nutrients. A diagnosis can be made by an upper endoscopy with biopsy.
Ulcerative colitis usually affects continuous stretches of the colon and rectum.
Whipple's disease is rare chronic disease caused by a bacterial infection. The affected bowel is usually swollen with raised, yellowish patches.

5. C: A positive Murphy's sign aids in the diagnosis of acute cholecystitis.

The Brudziński sign is positive when flexion of the neck usually causes flexion of the hip and knee. This maneuver is used to help diagnose meningitis.

The psoas sign is positive when a patient experiences abdominal pain when he or she actively flexes the leg at the hip and knee. This maneuver is used to help diagnose appendicitis.

The Levine sign is positive when a patient is holding a clenched fist over his or her chest to describe dull, pressing chest pain consistent with the discomfort of angina pectoris.

6. B: Vicryl sutures are absorbable. They take anywhere from 40 to 70 days to absorb. Other examples of absorbable sutures include Monocryl and chromic gut. Prolene, silk, and nylon sutures are all nonabsorbable sutures. Other examples of nonabsorbable suture materials include polyester sutures and stainless steel sutures. Dermabond is a type of skin adhesive meant for superficial skin lacerations; it should never be used on any other surface besides the skin.

7. C: Esophageal achalasia is when the lower esophageal sphincter does not relax properly. This impairs the smooth passage of food from the lower esophagus into the stomach. Acid reflux, dysphagia, and chest pain are symptoms of esophageal achalasia. Hematochezia is when a person has bright-red blood coming from the rectum. This occurrence is commonly associated with gastrointestinal (GI) bleeding.

8. C: CREST syndrome includes five main features: **c**alcinosis, **R**aynaud's syndrome, **e**sophageal dysmotility, **s**clerodactyly, and **t**elangiectasia. The CREST syndrome is part of the immune disorder scleroderma. This immune disorder causes skin and body tissues to improperly tighten.

Solar urticaria is the development of hives when the skin is exposed to sunlight; it is not related to CREST syndrome.

9. B: Reiter's syndrome causes inflammation of the urinary tract, eyes, skin, mucous membranes, and joints. Chlamydia is the most common cause of Reiter's syndrome.

Sjögren's syndrome is a disorder of the immune system that causes a decrease in the production of mucus and moisture.

Turner syndrome is a genetic condition in which females are missing all or part of an X chromosome. Some of the symptoms may include infertility, amenorrhea, short stature, and webbed neck.

Down syndrome is a genetic condition in which there is a chromosomal abnormality on chromosome 21. Some signs of Down syndrome may include broad forehead and tongue, slanted eyes, small ears, and cognitive and cardiac defects.

10. D: Ceftriaxone 250 mg IM injection in a single dose plus azithromycin 1 gm PO in a single dose or doxycycline 100 mg PO BID for seven days is the recommended regimen for treating gonorrhea (GC)/chlamydia infections. Clindamycin and Maxipime are not given as treatment for either gonorrhea or chlamydia. The patient should be treated in the ER for suspected GC/chlamydia infection to prevent the patient from potentially spreading the disease.

11. B: Naloxone (Narcan) is an opiate antidote to treat potential or confirmed narcotic overdoses. Oxycodone is an opiate.

Prednisolone is a corticosteroid drug. It is useful for the treatment of a wide range of inflammatory and autoimmune conditions.

Buspirone is used in the short-term relief of anxiety symptoms. Although this may be useful as a maintenance drug for the patient's history of anxiety, he is not anxious during the examination.

12. D: Augmentin is a penicillin, and cefepime and cephalexin are cephalosporins. Approximately 10% of patients with a penicillin reaction will also have an allergy to the cephalosporins. In patients with a documented allergy to pencillins, the use of cephalosporins is contraindicated. Clarithromycin is a macrolide and may be safely administered to a patient with a penicillin allergy.

13. A: Pegged teeth, also known as Hutchinson's teeth; swollen joints; deafness; blindness; and other nervous-symptom abnormalities are characteristic of congenital syphilis.
Down syndrome patients have a myriad of physical signs such as broad forehead and tongue, eyelid creases, small ears, short stature, and a flat head. They do not have pegged teeth and generally have unusually flexible joints.
Osgood–Schlatter disease is characterized by chronic knee pain in young children and adolescents.
Turner syndrome is a genetic condition in which females are missing all or part of an X chromosome. Some of the symptoms may include infertility, amenorrhea, short stature, and a webbed neck.

14. B: A hordeolum appears as a red, swollen, tender pimple on the edge of the eyelid. It is caused by an oil gland that has become blocked.
Xanthelasma are raised, yellow patches on the eyelids. The incidence of occurrence increases with age. They are common in patients with hyperlipidemia.
Mongolian spots are nonraised, grayish-blue skin lesions most commonly seen on the sacrum or buttocks.
A felon is an infection inside the fingertip that can expand and spread if left untreated.

15. D: Xanthelasma are raised yellow patches on the eyelids. The incidence of occurrence increases with age. They are common in patients with hyperlipidemia.
Dermoid cysts are skin growths or outpouchings that may contain miscellaneous structures such as skin, hair, or teeth. They are not skin lesions that develop over time; they are seen at birth.
Impetigo is a bacterial infection that is most commonly caused by *Staphylococcus aureus* or *Streptococcus pyogenes*. It causes lesions that can occur anywhere on the body. They are small, red, and pus-filled and can crack open and form a yellow or honey-colored, thick crust. They occur most commonly in young children.
Mongolian spots are flat, blue, or blue-gray skin markings near the buttocks that commonly appear at birth or shortly thereafter.

16. C: Medulloblastomas are the most common malignant brain tumor and are significantly more common in children than in adults. They usually occur in the cerebellum.
A hygroma is a collection of cerebrospinal fluid in the subdural space. Acute hygromas are usually caused by head trauma or a recent neurosurgical procedure.
Schistosomiasis is a chronic parasitic infection due to eating improperly cooked pork. On a magnetic resonance imaging (MRI) scan of the brain, it can appear as multiple enhancing nodules occurring on bilateral cerebral hemispheres.
Melanoma is a malignant skin cancer.

17. A: Charcot's triad is the combination of jaundice, fever, and right-upper quadrant abdominal pain. It occurs as a result of ascending cholangitis.
Acute appendicitis usually presents as periumbilical, epigastric, or right-lower quadrant abdominal pain, fever, nausea, vomiting, and extreme sensitivity to movement called the jar sign.
Choledocholithiasis is the presence of stones within the common bile duct without infection. Patients do not usually display symptoms.
Acute pyelonephritis usually presents as fever, shaking chills, epigastric or left-sided abdominal pain, nausea, vomiting, urinary tract infection (UTI) symptoms, and back pain.

18. C: In early pregnancy, high levels of estrogen cause increased venous pressure, causing the mucosal surfaces of the genitals to turn a purplish or bluish color.

The obturator sign is positive when abdominal pain is elicited with the internal rotation of the flexed right leg. This maneuver helps diagnose appendicitis.

The Levine sign is positive when a patient is holding a clenched fist over his or her chest to describe dull, pressing chest pain consistent with the discomfort of angina pectoris.

Kerning's sign is positive when a patient is unable to extend his or her leg when the hip is flexed. This maneuver helps diagnose meningitis.

19. A: Colchicine is used only in acute gout attacks.

Allopurinol (Zyloprim) is used for the treatment of chronic gout and is used to prevent rather than treat gout attacks. Other treatments for gout include nonsteroidal anti-inflammatory drugs (NSAIDs) and steroids. Tetracycline is an antibiotic and is not used to treat gout.

Amantadine has been used in the treatment of the influenza virus and for Parkinson's disease.

20. A: The Dix–Hallpike test involves a patient sitting upright with his or her head laterally rotated to one side. The patient is asked to lie down quickly with his or her head slightly extended. The test is considered positive if this maneuver reproduces symptoms.

An electroencephalogram (EEG) helps diagnose seizures or abnormal brain activity.

The transcranial Doppler ultrasound (TCD) measures the presence of vasospasm in the brain's blood vessels.

Phalen's maneuver is a diagnostic tool used to help diagnose carpal tunnel syndrome.

21. B: This child has Down syndrome, which is caused by a defect of chromosome 21.

Chromosome 23 is the sex chromosome.

Turner syndrome is a genetic condition in which females are missing all or part of an X chromosome. Some of the symptoms may include infertility, amenorrhea, short stature, and webbed neck.

Klinefelter's syndrome patients have an extra Y chromosome, leading to poor muscle strength, decreased fertility or infertility, gynecomastia, and low testosterone levels.

There is no chromosome 24. All humans have 23 chromosomal pairs, totaling 46 chromosomes.

Patients with abnormalities on chromosome 13 (also known as Patau's syndrome) usually have serious brain, pulmonary, and circulatory defects that are often fatal. Few patients survive infancy. Those that survive have severe intellectual and physical disabilities.

22. A: Electrical alternans is the alternation of the QRS complex between beats, most commonly seen with pericardial tamponade or severe pericardial effusion. Given the patient's history of recent surgery and his diagnosis of pericardial tamponade, this patient most likely has Dressler's syndrome. This can occur days to months after a cardiac injury when the body mistakenly attacks healthy heart tissue.

23. C: Severe ischemia can result in electrocardiogram (EKG) changes within minutes of the occurrence. Other helpful diagnostic aids would include troponin level, creatine phosphokinase-MB (CPK-MB) level, and a two-dimensional echocardiogram (2D echo). These aids can be more diagnostic than an EKG, but an EKG result is obtained much quicker than blood work or a 2D echo. It takes a minimum of three hours for a cardiac insult to be reflected in blood tests.

Choice a would show an anterior myocardial infarction (MI).

Choice b would show a lateral-wall MI.

Choice d would show a posterior-wall MI.

24. B: There are two types of second-degree heart block. (1) Mobitz type I (Wenckebach block) is characterized by progressive prolongation of the PR interval on beats followed by a blocked P wave/dropped QRS complex. The PR interval resets, and the cycle repeats.
(2) Mobitz type II heart block is characterized by intermittently nonconducting P waves. The PR interval remains unchanged.
In first-degree heart block, there is a prolonged PR interval that regularly precedes a QRS complex.
In third-degree heart block (complete heart block), there is no apparent relationship between P waves and QRS complexes.
Asystole is a state of no cardiac electrical activity.

25. A: The other modalities would be used if the patient had symptomatic bradycardia. Symptoms of bradycardia may include pallor, weakness, dizziness, altered mental status, fatigue, and shortness of breath. If the patient had been symptomatic, atropine is the first-line agent used. In the event that atropine is ineffective, epinephrine and dopamine may be used. If the patient displays signs of poor perfusion, he or she may be a candidate for transcutaneous pacing.

26. D: Hypertension is not a factor in Beck's triad. Beck's triad is the combination of distended jugular veins due to increased venous pressure, hypotension due to low arterial pressure, and muffled heart sounds due to excessive fluid on the heart. It occurs as a result of pericardial effusion. Aside from physical examination findings, an electrocardiogram (EKG) and/or a two-dimensional echocardiogram may help diagnose this condition.

27. C: Warm air does not commonly cause an asthma exacerbation, although extreme heat or humidity may cause an asthma attack. Cold air usually triggers an asthma attack because it can irritate the airways. Sinusitis or any upper respiratory infection that affects breathing can cause irritation and induce an asthma attack.
Cigarette smoke is a common trigger that can cause irritation and inflammation in the airways, which can aggravate asthma. Patients who live around tobacco smokers are predisposed to developing asthma. Allergens such as dust and pollen can aggravate the airways, which can induce an asthma attack.

28. B: The beta cells, which are located in the islets of Langerhans in the pancreas, secrete insulin. Insulin stimulates the cells to store glucose, lowering the blood sugar levels.
The alpha cells produce glucagon, which stimulates cells to break down their glucose reserves to raise the serum glucose level.
The gamma cells of the pancreas secrete a specialized type of peptide, which reduces one's appetite.
The delta cells of the pancreas secrete somatostatin, which plays a role in food absorption by the small intestine.

29. D: Diabetics are at risk for hypertension, not hypotension. Diabetics have higher levels of blood sugar because the pancreas produces insufficient or no insulin. High levels of blood glucose stimulate systemic inflammation and atherosclerosis formation, causing a multitude of other pathologies.
Atherosclerotic plaques decrease the lumen of blood vessels, causing hypertension. Excessive deposits in the renal tubules can cause chronic renal insufficiency and potentially renal failure.
The systemic inflammation caused by diabetes can also lead to neuropathy.

30. D: The most effective treatment of *Helicobacter pylori* is the combination of two antibiotics (amoxicillin, clarithromycin, metronidazole, and tetracycline) and a proton pump inhibitor. Two antibiotics are recommended due to potential antibiotic resistance. It is recommended that the patient be treated for 7 to 14 days to increase the chances of complete recovery.

31. A: Obesity is not a major risk factor.

More than half of the diagnosed cases of peptic ulcers are caused by *Helicobacter pylori.*

*H. pylori* may be diagnosed with a stool antigen test, a blood antibody test, and a carbon urea breath test, as well as other modalities.

Major risk factors include smoking, alcohol consumption, and nonsteroidal anti-inflammatory drug (NSAID) use.

32. D: Parkinson's disease destroys dopamine-producing neurons in the substantia nigra and causes motor symptoms (dyskinesia, tremor, rigidity) as well as cognitive symptoms. Approximately 80% of the substantia nigra is destroyed prior to the onset of symptoms.

Norepinephrine and epinephrine are major components in the body's fight-or-flight response.

Serotonin is involved with a multitude of functions including mood, cell growth, and hemostasis.

33. C: Parkinson's disease destroys dopamine-producing neurons in the substantia nigra and causes motor symptoms (dyskinesia, tremor, rigidity) as well as cognitive symptoms. Approximately 80% of the substantia nigra is destroyed prior to the onset of symptoms.

The medulla oblongata helps control the sympathetic and parasympathetic nervous systems, respirations, and basic reflexes.

The hippocampus plays a major role in storing old memories and the formation of new ones.

The pituitary gland controls major endocrine functions, pain relief, temperature regulation, and water balance. It is sometimes called the "master gland," because it is responsible for regulating so many important body functions.

34. C: Left bundle branch block acts as a red flag for four conditions: severe aortic valve disease, ischemic heart disease, chronic hypertension, and cardiomyopathy.

Pericardial tamponade generally has abnormalities with QRS complexes on electrocardiogram (EKG).

Pulmonary emboli are generally diagnosed by ventilation-perfusion (VQ) scan or computed tomography (CT) angiogram of the chest. In some patients with a pulmonary embolus, the EKG may be normal. The most common EKG findings are T-wave abnormalities.

Mitral valve prolapse is generally not diagnosed on an EKG. It is usually diagnosed by the patient's history, auscultation with a stethoscope, and two-dimensional echocardiogram.

35. B: This patient may have a pulmonary embolus, which is best diagnosed with a computed tomography (CT) angiogram of the chest. Sickle-cell disease increases the risk of pulmonary embolus, stroke, heart attack, pulmonary hypertension, skin ulcers, priapism, as well as other health problems.

A CT scan of the chest without contrast would most likely be nondiagnostic. Waiting for a troponin level or an arterial blood gas (ABG) would increase the risk of mortality in this patient.

36. A: The classic four features of tetralogy of Fallot include ventricular septal defect, narrowing of the pulmonary outflow tract, right ventricular hypertrophy, and an overriding aorta. Tetralogy of Fallot is the most common cyanotic heart defect. The reason why cyanosis occurs is due to the mixing of oxygen-rich and oxygen-poor blood through the ventricular septal defect.

37. A: The most common congenital heart defect is ventricular septal defect. The hole may be small and may spontaneously close on its own. If the hole is small but remains patent, the patient may be asymptomatic. If the hole is large enough to cause symptoms, it may warrant surgical intervention.

The occurrence of aortic stenosis increases with age, but it is not the most common heart defect.

Tricuspid atresia is one of the most uncommon cyanotic congenital heart defects.

Tetralogy of Fallot is the most common type of cyanotic congenital heart defect.

38. D: A persistent, dry cough is the most common side effect of taking angiotensin-converting enzyme (ACE) inhibitors. The development of a cough is not serious and does not have any long-term health complications. In the event that the cough persists, the patient should be placed on a different medication regimen. Switching to another ACE inhibitor would not be helpful because if one ACE inhibitor causes a cough, all medications of this class would likely cause the same symptom.

39. C: *Staphylococcus aureus* is a gram-positive coccus that is responsible for common skin infections as well as other illnesses.
*Staphylococcus pseudintermedius* is a gram-positive coccus. It is very common in animals, especially dogs, but it is rare in humans.
*Haemophilus influenzae* is a gram-negative coccobacillus. It is a main cause of pneumonia, meningitis, as well as other pathologies. It does not commonly cause skin infections.
*Streptococcus pneumoniae* is one of the main causative organisms in pneumonia, meningitis, as well as other pathologies. It is much less common in skin infections.

40. D: Addison's disease is caused by a lack of cortisol. Giving cortisol exogenously helps alleviate the disease's symptoms.
Diabetes is caused by insufficient or complete lack of insulin production. Many diabetic patients depend on insulin injections in order to help control their disease.
Patients with insufficient growth hormone depend on somatropin injections to help alleviate their disease's symptoms.
Synthroid (levothyroxine) is a medication taken by patients with hypothyroidism.

41. C: Hypotension plays no role in the pathology of chronic obstructive pulmonary disease (COPD). Because the lungs are chronically damaged, the patient is more predisposed to pulmonary infections such as pneumonia.
Cor pulmonale is right-sided heart failure caused by pulmonary hypertension. Because COPD is an obstructive disease that occurs in the lungs, it increases the right ventricle's afterload, which causes the ventricle to swell and become dilated. Perfusion becomes more strenuous, and the blood pressure increases to keep pace.
The risk of myocardial infarction increases in the presence of COPD because COPD causes heart failure, which can lead to a heart attack and potentially cardiac arrest.

42. B: Symptoms of cystic fibrosis (CF) may include abdominal discomfort from chronic constipation, salty-tasting skin, poor appetite, fatigue, fever, and pancreatitis. There are a myriad of signs and symptoms in patients with CF. A physical examination and medical history of both the child and the parents are important in making the diagnosis. The sweat chloride test is the standard diagnostic test for cystic fibrosis, but there are other modalities to test for CF, including genetic testing, stool tests, computed tomography (CT) scan of the chest, or a chest x ray.

43. B: Sickle-cell disease is an autosomal-recessive genetic blood disorder caused by a defect on chromosome 11. Patients who have only one recessive allele have sickle-cell trait; they are usually asymptomatic and do not suffer the same medical complications as those with the disease. Sickle-cell disease increases the risk of stroke, heart attack, pulmonary hypertension, skin ulcers, priapism, as well as other health problems. Sickle-cell disease does not increase the risk for diabetes.

44. D: The patient has a urinary tract infection and needs an antibiotic to cover gram-negative organisms. The most common cause of urinary tract infections is *Escherichia coli*. Augmentin would not provide sufficient coverage. Choices a and b would be used to treat potential gonorrhea (GC)/chlamydia

infections. Patients with urinary tract infections should be treated for a minimum of three days and up to seven days.

45. A: Macrobid is a category B medication, which are generally considered safe for use in pregnant women. The other choices are category C medications. Category C medications have shown potential adverse effects in prior research studies, but they may sometimes be used depending on the importance of the indication. Because the patient has a urinary tract infection (UTI), which is important, but not life-threatening, plus, she has no drug allergies, there are safer alternatives to use besides category C medications.

46. A: You should advise all patients with presumed or confirmed venereal disease to inform their partner(s) as soon as possible so they can also get tested. This helps to prevent others from spreading the disease and potentially infecting more people. As a medical provider, you cannot tell the patient's family or loved ones without permission without breaking Health Insurance Portability and Accountability Act (HIPAA) privacy laws.

47. B: Bipolar disorder is generally described as intermittent periods of mania and depression. Dysthymic disorder is a milder form of depression; there are no periods of mania. Posttraumatic stress disorder is described as feelings of stress, anger, anxiety, or depression after witnessing or experiencing a traumatic event. An adjustment disorder is described as having feelings of stress, anger, anxiety, or general emotional lability after experiencing a major life change such as moving away from home or starting a new school.

48. D: Pyridium is often given in conjunction with an antibiotic to help alleviate dysuria. The most common side effect of Pyridium is bright-orange urine. Other common side effects may include headache and rash. Although the decision to discontinue the medication must be based on the severity of the side effects, a change in urine color should not be the reason to discontinue the medication. The urine will go back to its normal color once the medication course has been completed.

49. C: Increasing one's fluid intake is the most important way to help prevent kidney stones. Kidney stones are usually made up of calcium oxalate, which can be found in dairy, fruits such as apples and grapes, vegetables such as broccoli and turnips, beer, as well as several other foods. Those who suffer from kidney stones may find it advisable to limit foods high in calcium oxalate.

50. B: Escitalopram is a serotonin reuptake inhibitor (SSRI) commonly used to treat anxiety and depression. Levothyroxine is a synthetic thyroid hormone medication used for those with hypothyroid disease. Amiodarone is used to treat cardiac arrhythmias such as atrial fibrillation and ventricular fibrillation. Haloperidol is an antipsychotic medication that can also be used to treat drug or alcohol withdrawal symptoms. Because this woman is not intoxicated and has no history of substance abuse or psychotic episodes, this medication would not be appropriate.

51. A: Von Willebrand disease is a hereditary bleeding disorder caused by factor VIII clotting deficiency. It is a much milder form of hemophilia. Thalassemia is a genetic disorder that causes an inadequate level of hemoglobin to be produced in the body, causing chronic anemia. Myeloma is a cancer of the plasma cells. It may present with anemia, but also with bone pain, infection, fatigue, and loss of bowel or bladder function. It is not affected or controlled by factor VIII.

52. C: Cauda equina syndrome can be caused by disease, trauma, or infection. It affects the nerve roots from L1 to L5 and S1 to S5, which can cause motor dysfunction, urinary retention, and saddle anesthesias,

- 61 -

among other neurological issues. It can be diagnosed with a computed tomography (CT) scan or magnetic resonance imaging (MRI) scan. A spine surgeon will decide whether or not the patient needs surgical decompression based on the presentation and radiological findings.

Kyphosis is a degeneration of the thoracic spine, causing a "hunchback" appearance.

Fibromyalgia is a disease causing chronic pain, which is potentially due to oversensitive nerves.

A Greenstick fracture is most commonly seen in children due to the flexibility of their bones. It occurs when the bony cortex bends abnormally, causing a partial break.

53. C: Slipped capital femoral epiphysis is when the femoral head is displaced from the acetabulum, causing hip and knee pain as well as gait disturbances. Once diagnosed, it is usually surgically corrected to prevent avascular necrosis of the femoral head. It is usually seen in prepubescent and pubescent children who are going through a growth spurt.

Osteitis pubis is a noninfectious inflammation of the pubic symphysis, causing lower abdominal or groin pain. This condition is normally seen in athletes.

Developmental dysplasia of the hip is when a child is born with one or both femoral heads spontaneously displaced from the acetabulum. This is diagnosed when the child is a toddler or when a young child is learning to walk.

Paget's disease is the abnormal formation and degeneration of bone usually in a localized area in the body. It is extremely uncommon in children.

54. D: Bisphosphonates such as Fosamax, nonsteroidal anti-inflammatory drugs (NSAIDs), and calcitonin are the mainstays of treatment for Paget's disease. Paget's disease is the abnormal formation and degeneration of bone, usually in a localized area of the body. Alkaline phosphatase is found in bone; after bony destruction or injury, it is released into the blood, increasing serum levels. It is one way to diagnose this disease. The diagnosis can also be made on CT scan, magnetic resonance imaging (MRI), or bone scan. Colchicine would provide little value because it is used to treat acute gout exacerbations.

55. B: Retinal artery occlusion is commonly caused by a clot that blocks the blood flow to the eye; it is very common in patients with coagulopathy disorders, hypertension, diabetes, or advanced atherosclerosis. The most common presentation is unilateral vision loss.

Conjunctivitis is the bacterial, viral, or allergy-induced inflammation of the conjunctiva, which may cause a foreign-body sensation, redness, visual disturbances, itching, tearing, and discharge. It does not cause sudden, painless blindness.

Acute angle closure glaucoma occurs when the intraocular pressure is so high that it damages the optic nerve, which could impair vision and cause severe eye pain. Patients usually note visual disturbances prior to actually losing their vision, such as seeing halos around objects. They may also present with headache on the same side as the vision loss, orbital or periorbital pain, nausea, and vomiting.

Retinal detachment is commonly caused by trauma, but it can also be caused by advanced age or disease processes such as diabetes. Immediately prior to losing vision, patients usually have partial vision loss or visual disturbances such as the appearance of flashes and floaters.

56. B: Using a tongue depressor to directly visualize the oropharynx is contraindicated in epiglottitis because this may induce airway spasm.

Direct visualization can be performed by an ear, nose, and throat (ENT) doctor after the patient is intubated and in the OR, so that the patient's airway is protected.

A lateral cervical spine x-ray may help confirm the suspected diagnosis; a thickened epiglottis often appears on x-ray as a "thumbprint sign."

Administration of penicillins, cephalosporins, or clindamycin is recommended.

57. B: Bacteria are the most common cause of otitis externa, or swimmer's ear. There are many bacterial pathogens, but *Pseudomonas aeruginosa* is the most common cause. *Staphylococcus aureus* and *Haemophilus influenzae* cause otitis externa as well, but they are not as common. *Aspergillus* is one of the most common fungal pathogens of otitis externa, along with *Candida albicans*. Fungal pathogens are more common in diabetic patients or those who are immunocompromised.

58. B: Antibiotic ear drops and pain medications are the mainstays of medical management of otitis externa.
Oral antibiotics are generally not prescribed.
Imaging of the brain or the ears is generally not indicated unless abscess or osteomyelitis is suspected; these complications are very rare.
An ear, nose, and throat (ENT) consult is not necessary for otitis externa. It is a very common condition, which usually resolves with antibiotics.

59. A: Labyrinthitis is the most likely diagnosis. It usually follows a viral infection such as the flu or the common cold, although it can occur after trauma or because of substance abuse. It differs from Ménière's disease because hearing and balance do not deteriorate after each episode. In cases of labyrinthitis, inner ear functions return to baseline after every episode. In Ménière's disease, there is a chronic deterioration of inner ear function.
Due to the patient's normal physical examination and vital signs, infectious processes such as otitis media and mastoiditis should be ruled out.

60. D: The patient has benign prostatic hypertrophy, which becomes more common in men as they age. Tamsulosin is an alpha-blocker, which improves urinary retention caused by benign prostate enlargement.
Terbinafine is used for tinea unguium.
Tramadol is an opiate medication used to alleviate pain.
Tegretol is used for the medical management of seizures.

61. A: The thiazolidinediones such as pioglitazone and sulfonylurea medications such as glimepiride and glyburide are pregnancy category C medications. Category C medications have shown potential adverse effects in prior research studies, but they may sometimes used depending on the importance of the indication. Medications such as Novolin are pregnancy category B medications, which should be used before trying a pregnancy category C medication, if possible. Because this patient has not yet had any medications for her diabetes, Novolin is the most preferable.

62. B: Although the patient is at risk for developing diabetes, his fasting blood sugar and hemoglobin A1C are normal. Medications at this point are unnecessary. Rechecking the hemoglobin A1C in one week would be useless because it is a calculation of an average blood sugar level over a three-month period. This patient's hemoglobin A1C doesn't need to be checked for at least another three months.

63. B: This woman should be checked when she is 38 years old. The current recommendation in the United States is to get screened 10 years prior to the age of a first-degree relative who was diagnosed with colon cancer. If no risk factors are present, then it is recommended to obtain a colonoscopy by 50 years of age. Because her father was 48 years old when he was diagnosed, she should get screened at age 38. If she had no significant family history, then her first colonoscopy should be when she is 50 years old.

64. C: Erythromycin helps shorten the course of the illness. It may also help prevent the child from spreading it to others if administered early enough. If erythromycin is given too late in the course of the

- 63 -

disease, it is ineffective. Augmentin, clindamycin, and guaifenesin play no role in the treatment or prevention of pertussis. The most important way to prevent pertussis is to get vaccinated.

65. C: The patient has respiratory syncytial virus (RSV). It is an acute, self-limiting, usually non-life-threatening virus that most commonly presents with a barking, or "seal-like," cough. It is more prevalent in children who attend day care, small children who live with school-aged children, and children who live in a home in which someone smokes.
The patient's fever and other presenting symptoms make asthma a less likely diagnosis.
Pneumonia usually presents with a high fever (above 101.5° F), productive cough, myalgias, shortness of breath, as well as a myriad of other symptoms. A barking cough is usually not present.
Patients with cystic fibrosis display signs and symptoms very early in life such as abdominal discomfort from chronic constipation, poor weight gain, steatorrhea, salty-tasting skin, poor appetite, fatigue, fever, and pancreatitis. It would not develop suddenly in a three-year-old child with no prior symptoms.

66. D: A primary, or spontaneous, pneumothorax occurs in the absence of underlying pulmonary pathology. The patient has no past medical history such as lung cancer or cystic fibrosis. A secondary, or complicated, pneumothorax occurs due to underlying pulmonary disease such as lung cancer, cystic fibrosis, chronic obstructive pulmonary disease (COPD), or other diseases. Trauma, such as a stab wound or a gunshot wound, can cause a pneumothorax, but there was no trauma noted in the physical examination or the medical history. Pneumonia may cause chest pain and shortness of breath, but there would not be an absence of lung markings on the chest x-ray. Lung cancer would show up as a radio-opaque mass or masses on chest x-ray.

67. B: This patient most likely has tuberculosis. Other symptoms of tuberculosis may include nausea, vomiting, anorexia, and fatigue.
Bronchitis and pneumothoraces do not present with cavitary lesions on chest x-ray.
Lung cancer may present with cavitary lesions on x-ray, but the acute onset of symptoms and type of symptoms that he has points more toward an infectious etiology.

68. A: Oxymetazoline hydrochloride is a nasal decongestant that may cause rhinitis medicamentosa or rebound nasal congestion. Patients should be advised to discard the medication after three to five days to prevent this from happening.
Benzonatate is an antitussive that does not cause rhinitis medicamentosa.
Ofloxacin are antibiotic eardrops used to treat infections of the ear canal.
Guaifenesin is an expectorant used to treat cough and chest congestion.

69. D: This patient should be given a baby aspirin for prophylaxis against potential future heart attacks and simvastatin for his hyperlipidemia. It is recommended that one's LDL level should be 100 to 130 if no risk factors are present and less than 100 if risk factors are present. His blood pressure, heart, rate, two-dimensional echocardiogram, and stress test are normal: prescribing antihypertensive medications such as metoprolol and amlodipine is unnecessary.

70. C: Pyloric stenosis commonly presents in neonates, but presentation of symptoms may start when the child is several months old. The chief symptoms are abdominal pain, dehydration, swollen abdomen, and, most notably, projectile vomiting. The narrowed pylorus may feel like a small mass in the epigastrium.
A Mallory–Weiss tear in the esophageal junction is usually seen in alcoholic patients. It is caused by persistent episodes of vomiting; however, any pathological process that causes forceful coughing or vomiting may cause a Mallory–Weiss tear.

Gastroesophageal reflux disease (GERD) and gastritis may cause abdominal discomfort and occasionally vomiting, but they would not cause projectile vomiting, failure to thrive, or be associated with an abdominal mass.

71. C: A Mallory–Weiss tear in the esophageal junction is usually seen in alcoholic patients caused by persistent episodes of vomiting; however, any pathological process that causes forceful coughing or vomiting may cause a Mallory–Weiss tear.
Pyloric stenosis commonly presents in neonates, but presentation of symptoms may start when the child is several months old. It does not suddenly present in the sixth decade of life.
Celiac sprue is an immune reaction that damages the lining of the small intestine and prevents it from absorbing important nutrients. It presents with nausea, vomiting, diarrhea, and abdominal pain, which occur after ingesting gluten products.
Whipple's disease is a bacterial infection of the bowel. It is a rare infection that presents with fever, abdominal pain, nonbloody vomiting, diarrhea, and arthralgias.

72. C: Esotropia is a condition in which one eye is normal and the other deviates medially.
Exotropia is a condition in which one eye is normal and the other eye deviates laterally.
Hypertropia is a condition in which one eye is normal and the other eye deviates upward. Hypotropia is a condition in which one eye is normal and the other eye deviates downward. All of these conditions fall under the general term "strabismus," which means an abnormal alignment of the eyes.

73. B: Bacterial conjunctivitis is an infection of the conjunctiva, causing one or both eyes to have a pinkish or reddish appearance. It is usually associated with fever, purulent discharge, and yellow-gold crusting of the eyelids and lashes. It is common among children and is highly contagious.
Viral conjunctivitis usually presents with clear discharge. Fever and crusting around the lids and lashes are much less common.
Allergic conjunctivitis presents with itchy watery eyes, sneezing, sniffling, clear rhinorrhea, and other allergy symptoms.
Dacryoadenitis is an infection of the eye due to a clogged tear duct, which can present with red eyes, pain, swelling of the medial aspect of the upper eyelid, and lymphadenopathy.

74. A: Erythromycin ointment is the drug of choice in a child with bacterial conjunctivitis.
Ciprofloxacin ointment can also be used to treat bacterial conjunctivitis, but the use of fluoroquinolones is contraindicated in children.
Trifluridine is used to treat keratitis caused by herpes simplex.
Famciclovir is used to treat keratitis caused by herpes zoster.

75. D: Niacin's most common side effect is flushing, which may be associated with pruritus. If these symptoms develop, the dosage may need to be adjusted, but the drug does not have to be discontinued. Simvastatin, atorvastatin, and rosuvastatin may cause pruritus, but they generally cause jaundice, not flushing. Other side effects of statin medications may include fever, abdominal pain, and arthralgias.

76. A: The patient is not in any respiratory distress, and he is not hypoxic. He most likely has a bacterial pneumonia, which requires po antibiotics.
The chest x-ray shows the infiltrate: a computed tomography (CT) scan of the chest exposes the patient to more radiation that he does not need.
If he had significant past medical problems or appeared toxic, then hospitalization and intravenous (IV) antibiotics may be needed. The diagnosis of pneumonia can be made based on physical examination, medical history, and possibly a chest x ray.
The patient does not need an arterial blood gas (ABG) because he is saturating 98% on room air.

77. A: Niacin may cause flushing or pruritus, but it should not be discontinued unless symptoms are severe. Niacin should originally be prescribed at the lowest dose possible to help prevent these symptoms; if the patient tolerates the dosage, it can always be titrated up. If flushing and pruritus do occur, patients can take medications such as Decadron and/or Benadryl. Nonsteroidal anti-inflammatory drugs (NSAIDs) taken prior to the niacin dose can help to minimize flushing.

78. A: The child has croup, which is most commonly caused by the parainfluenza virus. Antibiotics would be of little value. Steroids and/or epinephrine would be prescribed if the patient was in respiratory distress or had a prolonged course of illness. The mainstays of therapy in uncomplicated cases of croup are humidified air, rest, and maintaining adequate hydration.

79. B: Trimethoprim-sulfamethoxazole is the first-line treatment in patients with *Pneumocystis* pneumonia (PCP). Augmentin and gentamicin play no role in the treatment of this disease. Corticosteroids may be used in conjunction with an antibiotic to treat PCP, but they are not to be used as the sole treatment. Patients with a CD4 count of less than 200 are at risk for contracting PCP. PCP is one of the leading causes of death in acquired immunodeficiency syndrome (AIDS) patients.

80. D: Dietary restrictions are an important part of controlling the neurological complications that phenylketonuria (PKU) may cause. Patients with PKU are unable to break down phenylalanine, a common amino acid found in foods. Patients with PKU must strictly adhere to diets low in phenylalanine. If the diagnosis is not made early or if patients are not compliant with their dietary restrictions, complications such as hyperactivity, seizures, and intellectual disability may occur.
Ritalin and antiseizure medications such as Dilantin will be used after sequelae develop.
Routine blood work is of little value: once the diagnosis is made via blood test, there is no need to do routine blood work.

81. C: Hand washing is the most important measure in preventing communicable diseases.
Wearing a face mask may help, but it does not fully prevent against spreading diseases. If someone's hands are contaminated and he or she touches the mouth or eyes, wearing a face mask will not prevent the person from getting ill.
Wearing gloves is important, but the gloves may rip. If the gloves touch a contaminated surface and then touch someone's mouth or face, the gloves will not prevent against getting ill. Maintaining a sterile environment at all times is not plausible.

82. D: Pregnant women may eat fish and seafood as long as they are cooked thoroughly. Listeriosis is spread through contaminated food. Therefore, avoiding unpasteurized milk is recommended. It is also recommended to thoroughly wash produce, cook meat and fish prior to eating it and to limit processed foods such as hot dogs and deli meats during pregnancy. Hot dogs and deli meats may be contaminated after they are cooked and prior to being packaged. Pregnant women infected with *Listeria monocytogenes* may exhibit only mild symptoms, but this may result in the death of the fetus.

83. B: Immediately cleansing the wound is the number-one way to help prevent rabies. The rabies vaccine will prevent rabies, but it usually takes longer to obtain than it does to wash the wound. If the animal is caught, it would have to be tested for rabies prior to subjecting the bite victim to a series of vaccinations. Administration of antibiotics may be necessary if a secondary infection develops, but this would not be useful in preventing rabies from occurring.

84. A: Lotrimin cream helps treat fungal infections. Mites burrowing underneath the skin cause scabies infections. Topical creams such as permethrin can be used to treat infections. Pills are available for

- 66 -

persistent infections refractory to topical treatment. Washing clothing and linens in hot water and avoiding infected people are ways to help prevent the spread of infection.

85. D: The patient most likely has a kidney stone. An abdominal computed tomography (CT) scan or a kidney, ureter, and bladder (KUB) x-ray should be ordered to confirm the diagnosis. Costovertebral angle (CVA) tenderness is usually a sign of a kidney infection.
Hepatitis and cholecystitis are unlikely because they usually present with right-upper quadrant or right epigastric pain. Liver function tests are usually not normal in cases of acute infection. CVA tenderness is not present.
Appendicitis, like nephrolithiasis, presents with nausea, vomiting, fever, and chills, but the abdominal pain is usually present in the right-lower quadrant or right epigastrium. CVA tenderness is not present.

86. B: Hypervolemia is the least likely to cause cardiac arrest. There are 12 main causes of cardiac arrest (six H's and six T's): hypovolemia, hypoxia, hydrogen ions (acidosis), hyperkalemia, hypokalemia, hypothermia, toxins, tamponade, tension pneumothorax, thrombosis, thromboembolism, and trauma. Hypervolemia may increase the heart's preload, which may eventually lead to heart failure, but it is much less likely to cause a myocardial infarction.

87. B: The patient is displaying signs of acute appendicitis. Causing discomfort by shaking the bed or chair in which the patient is positioned is called the jar sign. Causing discomfort by flexing the right leg at the hip and the knee is called the psoas sign. The patient has discomfort during these maneuvers due to peritoneal irritation. These maneuvers help diagnose acute appendicitis and are not present in the other conditions listed.

88. D: The patient has acute meningitis. The triad of meningitis is photophobia, nuchal rigidity, and headache, although fever, nausea, vomiting, anorexia, and flulike symptoms are also common. The patient has a positive Brudziński's sign. The Brudziński sign is positive when flexion of the neck causes flexion of the hip and knee due to inflammation of the meninges.
A subarachnoid hemorrhage or migraine headache may present with headache, nausea, and vomiting, but the Brudziński sign would not be positive in the presence of a subarachnoid hemorrhage or a migraine headache.
Vestibulocerebellar syndrome is a progressive neurological disease in which patients show symptoms in early childhood.

89. A: The patient most likely has a pericardial tamponade. Pericardial tamponade is the abnormal collection of fluid that develops on the heart due to injury or prior disease, although the cause may be idiopathic. The patient's symptoms are consistent with Beck's triad. Beck's triad is the combination of hypotension, muffled heart sounds, and distended jugular veins.
A pneumothorax is much less likely. The patient is saturating 99% on room air, and his lungs sounds are equal bilaterally.
An aortic dissection usually presents with sharp, tearing chest pain that radiates to the back. Auscultation of the heart usually reveals a blowing murmur, not quiet heart sounds.
Stable angina is described as chest pain that is alleviated with rest.

90. A: In first-degree heart block, there is a prolonged PR interval that regularly precedes a QRS complex. There are two types of second-degree heart block. Mobitz type I, or Wenckebach block, is characterized by progressive prolongation of the PR interval on beats followed by a blocked P wave/dropped QRS complex. The PR interval resets, and the cycle repeats.
Mobitz type II heart block is characterized by intermittently nonconducting P waves. The PR interval remains unchanged.

In third-degree (complete) heart block, there is no apparent relationship between P waves and QRS complexes.

91. C: Bulimia nervosa is a psychiatric disorder that usually occurs in female adolescents and young women that consists of forcefully purging after every meal in order to control one's weight. Signs and symptoms of this disorder are varied, but dental problems are most common due to the frequent exposure to stomach acid due to vomiting. Women who have this disorder are usually mildly overweight, or their weight is normal.
Dysthymic disorder is a milder form of depression.
Anorexia nervosa is when someone purposely severely limits his or her food intake in order to control his or her weight.
Panic disorder occurs when someone experiences extreme nervousness or fear that may or may not be connected to a specific trigger.

92. A: Haloperidol is an antipsychotic medication. This patient most likely has schizophrenia. Schizophrenia is a mental disorder that makes it hard for a person to differentiate between what is real and not real. It also affects one's concentration, mood balance, sleep, and ability to maintain appropriate behavior.
Choices b and c are selective serotonin reuptake inhibitors (SSRIs), which are used to treat anxiety, depression, panic disorder, and posttraumatic stress disorder. They may provide some relief of symptoms, but they should be used in conjunction with other antipsychotic medications.
Choice d is a sedative. This may provide some relief of symptoms, but it should not be the only medication used in a schizophrenic patient.

93. C: The child most likely has glucose-6-phosphate dehydrogenase (G6PD) deficiency. It is an X-linked recessive hereditary disease in which the defect of this enzyme causes red blood cells to break down prematurely. It is much more prevalent in males than females. It is the most common enzyme defect in humans. Many types of foods (such as legumes and artificial food coloring), medications (nonsteroidal anti-inflammatory drugs [NSAIDs], aspirin, and sulfa drugs), as well as environmental triggers (mothballs, pollen, and henna), can cause acute exacerbations. The only treatment for this disease is to avoid known triggers as much as possible.
Leukocytosis is the elevation of a person's white blood cell (WBC) count in the presence of infection, disease, or stress. The patient's WBC count is normal.
Thrombocytopenia is the presence of an abnormally low platelet count due to infection, medications (i.e., chemotherapy drugs), disease, or blood loss.
Von Willebrand disease is a hereditary bleeding disorder caused by factor VIII clotting deficiency. It is a much milder form of hemophilia. It doesn't cause jaundice or hemolytic anemia.

94. C: The mainstays of treatment for thalassemia major are folate supplements and regular blood transfusions. In cases of severe disease, chelation therapy (removal of excess iron from the blood) and bone marrow transplants are necessary. Thalassemia major is a rare genetic blood disorder in which the hemoglobin is defective and causes mild to severe hemolytic anemia. Patients with thalassemia should avoid iron because they are already at risk for iron overload in their blood due to regular blood transfusions.
Avoiding legumes, nonsteroidal anti-inflammatory drugs (NSAIDs), and henna would be suggestions for those with G6PD deficiency, not those who have thalassemia major.

95. D: This woman most likely has placenta previa, which commonly presents with painless, bright-red vaginal bleeding in the end of the second trimester or the beginning of the third trimester. It is due to a

low-lying placenta. As the uterus enlarges, it may push up against the placenta, causing a small part to tear, and bright-red bleeding occurs.

Placental abruption (abruptio placentae) is the complete separation of the placenta, causing bright-red vaginal bleeding, abdominal and/or back pain, and severe contractions.

Premature rupture of the membranes is when a woman's water breaks prior to the onset of labor. Dystocia is defined as difficult childbirth.

96. B: This woman may have an ectopic pregnancy versus a threatened abortion. Because she is only six weeks pregnant, the intrauterine pregnancy (IUP) may be too small to see. If the repeat beta human chorionic gonadotropin (HCG) increases normally and an IUP is seen after two days, then the diagnosis is most likely threatened abortion. If the beta HCG levels become higher than normal and an IUP still cannot be seen, then methotrexate or a surgical consult may be needed to treat the ectopic pregnancy.

97. A: Impetigo is a bacterial infection that is most commonly caused by *Staphylococcus aureus* or *Streptococcus pyogenes*. It causes lesions that can occur anywhere on the body. They are small, red, and pus-filled and can crack open and form a yellow or honey-colored, thick crust. They most commonly occur in young children. These lesions are contagious, and family members and friends should avoid touching them until they are completely healed. Family members should wash bed linens in hot water and avoid sharing personal-care products such as razors and towels with the patient to prevent the spread of the disease. Hand washing is strongly recommended as well.

98. B: Tinea corporis, also known as "ringworm," is a fungal infection that can occur anywhere on the body. It is usually described as a red, circular lesion with a central clearing with grayish or flesh-toned scales. Ketoconazole is an antifungal medication that is used to treat superficial fungal or yeast infections. Erythromycin, mupirocin, and metronidazole are all antibiotics used to treat bacterial infections. They are generally ineffective at treating fungal infections.

99. C: Paraphimosis is when the foreskin cannot be brought back to its original position. If it cannot be resolved at the bedside with conservative methods, then surgical intervention may be necessary. Cryptorchidism is a condition in which one or both testicles have not descended into the scrotum. Phimosis is when the foreskin cannot be retracted.

A hydrocele is the collection of fluid around the testicle due to infection or malignancy. Sometimes, the cause can be idiopathic.

100. D: Cryptorchidism usually resolves on its own without treatment. Because the child is so young, no intervention would be necessary at this time. If after one year of age the testicle still has not descended, then hormone injections may be necessary. If that fails, then an orchiopexy is needed. An undescended testicle carries an increased risk of developing testicular cancer and infertility.

101. A: A hydrocele is the collection of fluid around the testicle due to infection or malignancy. Sometimes, the cause can be idiopathic. It is not harmful and has no serious long-term complications.

Testicular torsion is a medical emergency. It occurs when the spermatic cord becomes twisted and blood flow to the testicle is severely diminished or absent. It presents with acute onset of pain and swelling of the affected testicle.

A varicocele is an enlargement of the veins in the scrotum, causing testicular aching and/or swelling to occur. The venous enlargement is usually due to faulty valves in the veins or compression of a neighboring vein disrupting blood flow in nearby veins.

Cryptorchidism is a condition in which one or both testicles have not descended into the scrotum.

102. D: A D-dimer test is a highly sensitive but nonspecific blood test for detecting the presence of clots. If the person is already diagnosed with a pulmonary embolus (PE), then the D-dimer will be positive. It will take weeks to months to get the clot to dissolve. Because the patient has sickle-cell disease and is at high risk for developing future clots, placing her on a heparin infusion, sending her home on warfarin, and placing an inferior vena cava (IVC) filter are viable treatment options. Because the patient has a PE that is causing chest pain, administering analgesics would be appropriate management.

103. C: He should be getting the influenza vaccine every year. Though he is not in a high-risk group (i.e., very young, very old, health-care worker, or immunocompromised), the vaccine still provides modest protection against contracting the influenza virus. Conservative measures such as frequent hand washing are also recommended. His tobacco abuse increases the risk of contracting pulmonary diseases such as influenza and also raises the complication rates in the event that he does contract the disease. Therefore, severely limiting tobacco use or quitting altogether is recommended.

104. B: Furosemide is used to treat congestive heart failure and edema, but it is not a treatment used in atrial fibrillation.
Metoprolol is a beta-blocker that helps slow the heart rate down.
Warfarin is a blood thinner that helps prevent the heart from sending clots to the lungs or brain.
Lanoxin reduces strain on the heart and is used to treat hypertension, cardiomyopathy, and atrial fibrillation.

105. D: Coccidioidomycosis, also known as "valley fever," is a self-limiting respiratory infection caused by a fungus endemic to southwestern soil in the United States. It may present with cough with or without hemoptysis and flulike symptoms. It may also present with erythema nodosum, which is painful erythematous lumps.
*Pneumocystis* pneumonia usually occurs in immunocompromised patients such as those with HIV. Symptoms are similar to the influenza virus. Patients most commonly have a nonproductive cough. The symptoms do not spontaneously resolve; po and sometimes IV antibiotics are needed to treat this opportunistic infection.
Symptoms of tuberculosis may include fever, night sweats, hemoptysis, nausea, vomiting, anorexia, and fatigue. This disease does not go away on its own.
Respiratory syncytial virus (RSV) is an acute, self-limiting, usually non-life-threatening virus that most commonly presents with a barking or "seal-like" cough. It is more prevalent in children who attend daycare, small children who live with school-aged children, and children who live in a home in which someone smokes.

106. A: A two-dimensional echocardiogram can make a definitive diagnosis of ventricular septal defect (VSD). VSD is the most common congenital heart defect. Smaller defects may close spontaneously, and no further treatment is needed. Larger defects can cause heart failure and pulmonary hypertension, as well as other complications.
A chest x-ray may show cardiomegaly, but it is not a definitive test of VSD.
An electrocardiogram (EKG) may show left ventricular hypertrophy, but it is not used as a definitive test for VSD.
Auscultation with a stethoscope may reveal a heart murmur, but it is not a dependable diagnostic aid for VSD.

107. B: Coarctation of the aorta is an acyanotic congenital heart defect commonly associated with Turner syndrome. Generally, it is more common in boys than girls. It involves a narrowing of the aorta, which may cause no symptoms depending on the severity of the narrowing. Symptoms can include syncope, chest pain, shortness of breath, dizziness, cold lower extremities, failure to thrive, and chronic fatigue. A

- 70 -

chest x ray may reveal the "figure 3 sign": prestenotic dilatation of the aortic arch and left subclavian artery, indentation at the coarctation, and poststenotic dilatation of the descending aorta.

108. C: Torsades de pointes literally means "twisting of the points." It is a polymorphic ventricular tachycardia that can be caused by congenital disease, electrolyte abnormalities caused by malnourishment or alcoholism, or adverse drug interactions. Administering antiarrhythmic medications and reversing the electrolyte abnormalities, if applicable, are the mainstays of therapy.

109. A: Prinzmetal's angina is a condition that typically occurs in young women. It is much more common in people who smoke cigarettes. It is due to vasospasm of coronary arteries; it spontaneously resolves without treatment. Typically, it will occur at rest, and no electrocardiogram (EKG) changes may be seen unless the test is performed during an acute episode.
Unstable angina is a condition in which chest pain occurs at rest and during activity due to severe atherosclerosis.
Stable angina is chest pain that is alleviated with rest due to mild to moderate atherosclerotic disease.
Costochondritis occurs when the chest wall is strained due to strenuous physical activity, trauma, or idiopathic cause. Palpation reproduces symptoms.

110. D: Small-cell carcinoma is responsible for causing a number of paraneoplastic syndromes such as syndrome of inappropriate antidiuretic hormone (SIADH), Cushing's syndrome, and limbic encephalitis. Paraneoplastic syndromes are a localized or systemic response to the presence of tumor cells in the body. The other three choices are subtypes of non-small-cell carcinoma, which is not commonly a cause of paraneoplastic syndromes.

111. C: A chest x-ray may be ordered in a case of infective endocarditis, but it is one of the least helpful tests compared to the other choices. A chest x ray may show cardiomegaly or a pyogenic abscess, but it can also be normal is some cases.
Blood cultures would be positive, which shows that the patient has bacteremia. An infection needs to be present in order to make the diagnosis of infective endocarditis.
A computed tomography (CT) scan of the chest would show a fluid collection, abscess, or inflammation around the endocardium.
An echocardiogram would show one or more vegetations on the heart; this is the preferred diagnostic aid.

112. C: Limiting one's tobacco use (or preferably quitting smoking altogether), limiting sodium intake, and increasing physical activity are all recommendations a health-care professional should make to a patient with prehypertension. Prehypertension is defined as systolic blood pressure of 120 to 139 and diastolic blood pressure 81 to 89 on three consecutive visits four to six weeks apart. Medication regimens can be avoided if patients take conservative measures to lower their blood pressure.

113. C: No intervention is needed. The patient has mitral valve prolapse, a condition in which the mitral valve does not close completely. In the majority of patients, mitral valve prolapse does not adversely affect their health and no intervention is needed. Some patients may experience chest pain, dizziness, palpitations, and dyspnea, and in these cases, further workup and possible intervention may be warranted.

114. B: The main treatment in the presence of a non-ST segment elevation myocardial infarction (NSTEMI) is oxygen, aspirin, nitroglycerin, and a beta-blocker if hypertension is present. Beta-blockers such as metoprolol decrease the workload of the heart. Antiplatelet medications, such as aspirin, are used to help prevent clot formation. Clopidogrel is used if aspirin is not tolerated, but in most situations, aspirin is the first-line antiplatelet regimen. Nitroglycerin helps increase the serum nitric oxide in the

- 71 -

blood, which helps prevent against further cardiac damage. A troponin level, an echocardiogram, and morphine may be administered once the patient has been stabilized.

115. A: This patient has stable angina. Stable angina is present when a patient experiences chest pain that is alleviated with rest. This condition occurs with mild to moderate atherosclerotic disease. A patient may develop chest pain during periods of physical activity caused by cardiac ischemia. During rest, the body's demands on the heart lessen and the blood flow becomes adequate enough to perfuse the heart. Prinzmetal's angina is a condition that typically occurs in young women in the presence or absence of atherosclerosis. It is much more common in people who smoke. It is due to vasospasm of coronary arteries; it spontaneously resolves without treatment. Typically, it will occur at rest. Unstable/variant angina is a condition in which chest pain occurs at rest and during activity due to severe atherosclerosis.
An aortic aneurysm is an outpouching of part of the vessel wall, or it may be a circumferential outpouching of the vessel wall caused by disease or trauma. Patients may be asymptomatic, but as the aneurysm becomes significantly large or ruptures, the patient will display severe abdominal or back pain. Symptoms do not resolve with rest.

116. B: Macular degeneration is an age-related eye disease that affects central vision, while peripheral vision is preserved. Approximately one-third of patients older than age 75 suffer from this condition. The macula is responsible for central vision; it is located on the center of the retina. Once macular degeneration occurs, there are some medications and dietary modifications that can slow the progression. It generally does not lead to blindness.
Open-angle glaucoma presents with worsening unilateral or bilateral painless blindness.
Acute-angle closure glaucoma occurs when the intraocular pressure is so high that it damages the optic nerve, which could impair vision and cause severe eye pain.
A clot blocking blood flow to the eye causes retinal artery occlusion; it is very common in patients with coagulopathy disorders, hypertension, diabetes, or advanced atherosclerosis.
The most common presentation is sudden unilateral vision loss.
Optic neuritis is the inflammation of the optic nerve due to infectious or immunologic disorders. It presents with sudden onset eye pain and loss of vision.

117. D: The patient may have an acoustic neuroma; a magnetic resonance imaging (MRI) scan of the brain is an essential diagnostic tool. Acoustic neuromas are tumors of the acoustic nerve that may cause facial droop or unilateral facial paresthesias/pain, ataxia, tinnitus, hearing loss, dizziness, and receptive aphasia.
An electromyography (EMG) test might be considered if muscle weakness or facial droop is present to test the activity of muscles and the nerves. This patient's physical examination is normal, so an EMG is of little use.
An ear, nose, and throat (ENT) consult would be appropriate once a workup has been done and tests have been resulted.
The Dix–Hallpike maneuver helps to confirm the diagnosis of benign positional vertigo. Movement does not exacerbate the patient's symptoms, so this condition should not be a differential diagnosis.

118. D: The child has aspirated her toy, and a stat bronchoscopy should be performed to confirm the diagnosis and remove the object.
If the child is stable, a chest x ray should be ordered to help confirm the diagnosis; however, in the presence of stridor and mild hypoxia, a bronchoscopy should be the first choice.
A blind finger sweep should be avoided because it may push the object further into the airway.
Although oxygen administration is recommended, nebulizer treatments would provide little added value; the child's respiratory distress is due to choking, not due to bronchospasm caused by disease.

- 72 -

119. B: The patient has a right-sided pleural effusion, most likely due to her chronic obstructive pulmonary disease (COPD). It is a pathologic fluid collection in the pleura. It may develop postoperatively, but more commonly it is caused by infection or disease. Pleural effusions may present with dyspnea, pleuritic chest pain, fever, and cough. In instances of a large pleural effusion, breath sounds will be diminished due to the fluid collection in the lung. Tactile fremitus is decreased due to the fluid in the pleural space, which decreases the lung's ability to expand. There is dullness to percussion due to the increased fluid and decreased air space.

In cases of a pneumothorax, the symptoms may present the same as those with pleural effusion. On physical examination, tactile fremitus is decreased due to the decreased lung space/size. Percussion is hyperresonant due to the extra air in the pleural space. Breath sounds are diminished.

Acute asthma exacerbation and influenza may present with similar symptoms, but there would be no decreased tactile fremitus or dullness to percussion.

120. B: The McMurray test is a maneuver that can help diagnose a meniscal tear. If you suspect a medial meniscal tear, place one hand on the patient's foot and another on the medial aspect of the affected knee. Flex the knee while internally rotating the leg. If you feel a pop or a click, and the patient experiences pain, the test is positive for meniscal injury. To diagnose a lateral tear, place one hand on the lateral aspect of the affected knee and externally rotate the leg.

The Murphy test helps to diagnose acute cholecystitis.

McBurney point tenderness helps diagnose acute appendicitis.

The obturator test helps diagnose acute appendicitis.

121. A: An avulsion fracture is when one piece of bone is separated from the whole.

A Greenstick fracture is most commonly seen in children due to the flexibility of their bones. It occurs when the bony cortex bends abnormally, causing a partial break.

A comminuted fracture is when the bone is shattered into several pieces.

An oblique fracture is a diagonal break in the bone.

122. A: This patient most likely has pneumoconiosis, also known as "miner's lung" due to a miner's prolonged coal-dust exposure. It presents as an upper respiratory infection that does not resolve. The honeycomb appearance on chest x-ray is a common finding. There is no medical treatment other than to remove the causative agent.

Schistosomiasis is a chronic parasitic infection caused by eating improperly cooked pork. On a magnetic resonance imaging (MRI) scan of the brain, it appears as multiple enhancing nodules occurring in bilateral cerebral hemispheres.

Tuberculosis is a bacterial infection of the lungs, causing symptoms such as night sweats, lymphadenopathy, fever, chills, hemoptysis, nausea, vomiting, anorexia, and fatigue.

Coccidioidomycosis, also known as "valley fever," is a self-limiting respiratory infection caused by a fungus endemic to soil of the southwestern United States. It may present with cough with or without hemoptysis and flulike symptoms. It may also present with erythema nodosum, which is characterized by painful erythematous lumps.

123. B: Testicular carcinomas present as hard, painless, fixed, solid testicular lesions. Your next step should be to order imaging studies and blood work to confirm the diagnosis.

A hydrocele is a soft, painless, fixed testicular mass. It is due to a collection of fluid around the testicle due to infection or malignancy. Sometimes, the cause is unknown. Hydroceles are not harmful and have no serious long-term complications.

A varicocele is an enlargement of the veins in the scrotum, causing testicular aching and/or swelling to occur. The venous enlargement is usually due to faulty valves in the veins or compression of a neighboring vein disrupting blood flow in nearby veins.

Testicular torsion is a medical emergency. It occurs when the spermatic cord becomes twisted, and blood flow to the testicle is severely diminished or absent. It presents with acute onset of pain and swelling of the affected testicle.

124. D: The drop-arm test can help confirm the diagnosis of a rotator cuff tear, although the only way to truly confirm the diagnosis would be a magnetic resonance imaging (MRI) scan. The examiner will have the patient abduct both arms 90° and rotate his arms so that the thumbs are pointing downward. If the patient is unable to keep his affected arm abducted when the examiner applies pressure, the examiner should suspect a rotator cuff tear. The other three maneuvers are helpful in diagnosing meniscus tears.

125. C: Mastoiditis is an infection of the mastoid bone of the skull. It is generally a complication of inner ear infections. Symptoms may include fever, ear pain, ear discharge, fever, swelling behind the ear (where the mastoid bone is located), hearing loss, headache, and erythema. Imaging studies such as magnetic resonance imaging (MRI) and computed tomography (CT) scans can make the definitive diagnosis.

Ménière's disease is a usually chronic disorder of the inner ear, causing a mild to severe sensation of fullness in the affected ear, vertigo, dizziness, and hearing loss. The exact cause is unknown, but it is most likely multifactorial. Ménière's disease is much more common in adults than in children. It does not cause fever or swelling behind the ear.

Acoustic neuromas are tumors of the acoustic nerve. They are much more common in adults than in children. Symptoms include hearing loss, dizziness, headache, tinnitus, facial droop, and ataxia. They do not cause fever or swelling behind the ear.

A cholesteatoma is a fluid-filled cyst, which may or may not be infected, caused by poorly functioning Eustachian tubes. Symptoms may include ear drainage, pain, and tinnitus. If infection is present, fever may occur as well. It does not cause swelling behind the ear.

126. C: *Cryptococcus* is the pathogen causing this patient's meningitis. It is one of the defining opportunistic infections of patients with acquired immunodeficiency syndrome (AIDS); their CD4 count is usually less than 200. It is the most common fungal pathogen in immunocompromised patients, such as those with cancer or AIDS. Diagnosis is made via India ink stain. Treatment includes po and/or IV antifungal medications. The prognosis for AIDS patients with *Cryptococcus* meningitis is very poor. The other choices provided are not diagnosed with an India ink stain.

127. A: Singulair is a leukotriene inhibitor. It is used to help prevent asthma exacerbations and seasonal allergies. It is a preventative medicine, but it should not be used as treatment during acute episodes. Singulair, Xopenex, and Ventolin are short-acting beta-2 bronchodilators. These medications are some of the first-line agents in treating an acute asthma exacerbation.

128. C: Wilms' tumor is the most common renal tumor in pediatric patients. The exact cause is unknown, but incidence does increase with family history, suggesting there is a genetic component. Symptoms may include abdominal pain, abdominal mass, nausea, vomiting, constipation, and changes in urine color. Signs such as hemihypertrophy and aniridia (complete or partial absence of the iris) may be associated with this disease.

Kaposi's sarcoma generally appears as multiple cutaneous lesions, but it may affect the internal organs as well.

Hodgkin's lymphoma is a malignancy of the white blood cells.

A lipoma is a benign tumor created by the overgrowth of fatty tissue.

129. B: Hyaline membrane disease, also known as infant respiratory distress syndrome, is a common cause of respiratory distress in premature infants. It is due to insufficient surfactant. Treatments include supplemental oxygen and the administration of synthetic surfactant.

*Pneumocystis* pneumonia usually occurs in immunocompromised patients. Symptoms are similar to the influenza virus. Patients most commonly have a nonproductive cough.

Pneumoconiosis, also known as "miner's lung," is a lung disease caused by prolonged dust exposure. Respiratory syncytial virus (RSV) is an acute, self-limiting, usually non-life-threatening virus that most commonly presents with a barking, or "seal-like" cough. It is prevalent in children who attend daycare, small children who live with school-aged children, and children who live in a home in which someone smokes.

130. C: This patient most likely has a hyphema, considering his symptoms and history of recent trauma. A hyphema is a localized hemorrhage in the eye due to rupture of the blood vessel(s).

A hordeolum appears as a red, swollen, tender pimple on the edge of the eyelid. It is caused by a blocked oil gland.

Optic neuritis is the inflammation of the optic nerve due to infectious or immunologic disorders. It presents with sudden-onset eye pain and loss of vision.

Blepharitis is the inflammation and swelling of the eyelid due to allergies, infection, or underlying conditions such as rosacea.

131. A: Leukoplakia is a condition in which white patches may develop on the tongue or inside the mouth. It is similar in appearance to oral thrush, except that in cases of thrush, the white lesions may be scraped off. The causes of leukoplakia are unknown, but it is commonly seen in alcoholics and those who smoke or chew tobacco.

Thrush is a yeast infection seen in patients who are poorly controlled diabetics, those who have been on long-term steroids or antibiotics, and immunocompromised patients.

Parotitis is an infection of the parotid gland, which can produce facial swelling and pain.

Gingivostomatitis is a yeast infection of the mouth and gums, appearing as painful sores.

132. D: Out of the choices given, tetralogy of Fallot is the only cyanotic congenital cardiac defect. It is the most common congenital cyanotic heart defect, usually associated with chromosomal abnormalities. Tetralogy of Fallot is most commonly caused by infections during pregnancy or by excessive alcohol intake during pregnancy. The radiological sign "boot-shaped heart" or "cœur en sabot" is most commonly associated with tetralogy of Fallot. The heart looks like a boot due to right-ventricular hypertrophy and pulmonary stenosis.

133. B: Bronchoscopy with biopsy would provide definitive confirmation of the diagnosis. Patients with sarcoidosis have multiple granulomas in their lungs as well as other organs. Sarcoidosis is a systemic inflammatory disease that can attack any organ, but it most commonly attacks the lymph nodes and lungs. A lumbar puncture would provide no diagnostic value.

A computed tomography (CT) scan and serum phosphorus may aid in the diagnosis, but they are not definitive tests.

134. C: This patient most likely has fibrocystic breast disease. It is a benign condition in which singular or multiple breast cysts develop. They can occur right before one's menses begins or may be unrelated to menses. People placed on hormone replacement therapy or birth control pills generally have less severe symptoms.

Breast cancer is unlikely, considering the patient's presentation and physical examination. Malignant breast masses don't shrink in size spontaneously, are generally nontender, and usually do not occur bilaterally.

- 75 -

Fibroadenomas are generally singular, rubbery, nontender breast lesions that are benign in nature. Gynecomastia is the appearance of breasts in males due to enlarged mammary glands. This may be due to obesity, congenital etiology, endocrine abnormality, or underlying disease. This condition usually resolves on its own in a patient with no significant past medical history.

135. A: A fibroadenoma is a benign breast mass that usually does not cause pain. It can be monitored; no intervention is necessary unless it becomes large and the patient requests removal.
Birth control pills are not useful in treating fibroadenomas.
Repeating a biopsy would not be helpful. Fibroadenomas are benign lesions that do not become malignant.
There is no reason for a mastectomy because fibroadenomas are benign lesions.

136. A: Clindamycin is not a medication that would be used in the treatment of tuberculosis. There are a multitude of medications used to treat tuberculosis; they are used in a variety of combination therapies. The more common medications are isoniazid, rifampin, pyrazinamide, and ethambutol. Less common drug remedies include amikacin, ethionamide, moxifloxacin, para-aminosalicylic acid, and streptomycin. Affected patients are usually on multiple medications for six months or longer.

137. D: Ascending or descending quickly will exacerbate the effects caused by barotrauma. Barotrauma is when the pressure in the middle ear is higher than that of the outer ear. Symptoms can include ear pain, hearing loss, and dizziness. The goal of treatment or prevention is to keep the Eustachian tubes open so the pressure between the outer ear and the inner ear remains normalized. Actions such as chewing gum, yawning, or sucking on candy can help keep the pressures normalized.

138. B: Bronchiolitis is a common viral upper respiratory infection in children. It usually starts with mild symptoms similar to those of the common cold and then progresses to wheezing, fever, breathing difficulties causing intercostal retractions, and in extreme cases, cyanosis due to respiratory insufficiency. Symptoms of tuberculosis may include fever, night sweats, hemoptysis, nausea, vomiting, anorexia, and fatigue.
Cystic fibrosis is a chromosomal disorder that causes the lungs to become chronically plugged with mucus. Symptoms may include abdominal discomfort from chronic constipation, salty-tasting skin, poor appetite, fatigue, fever, delayed growth, poor weight gain, clay-colored stools, and frequent episodes of pneumonia. The diagnosis is usually made before or shortly after the child is born.
Hyaline membrane disease, also known as infant respiratory distress syndrome, is a common cause of respiratory distress in premature infants. It is due to insufficient surfactant. Treatments include supplemental oxygen and the administration of synthetic surfactant.

139. B: Levothyroxine is a synthetic thyroid hormone used to treat Hashimoto's thyroiditis, which causes hypothyroidism.
Lanoxin is an antiarrhythmic agent used to treat conditions such as atrial fibrillation.
Lamisil is medication used to treat fungal infections.
Lantus is a type of exogenous insulin used to treat patients with diabetes.

140. D: Huntington's disease is a progressive neurological disorder caused by an autosomal-dominant chromosomal abnormality. It most commonly occurs in people between 30 and 40 years of age.
Tourette syndrome is first noticed in childhood and is characterized by involuntary verbal sounds or motor movements. It does not cause cognitive impairment, although it may be seen in the presence of cognitive disorders.
Guillain–Barré syndrome is an autoimmune disease that causes muscle weakness or paralysis; it does not cause cognitive impairment.

Cerebral palsy is a neurological disorder that causes motor and cognitive impairment. It is diagnosed in infancy or childhood. It may be caused by infection or trauma, but the most common cause is prenatal hypoxia.

141. C: This patient is suffering from hyperparathyroidism. Elevated serum calcium can cause a multitude of nonspecific symptoms such as weakness and fatigue, depression, bone pain, myalgias, constipation, polyuria, polydipsia, cognitive impairment, kidney stones, and osteoporosis.
Hypothyroidism causes a slowing in metabolism and potentially impaired cognitive function, producing symptoms as unintentional weight gain, low blood pressure, bradycardia, weakness, myxedema, and slow speech.
Hyperthyroidism causes an increase in metabolism, producing symptoms such as unintentional weight loss, high blood pressure, tremor, palpitations, and weakness.
Hypoparathyroidism will also cause many nonspecific symptoms; the most common is perioral and extremity paresthesias.

142. A: Permethrin cream is an insecticide used to treat skin infections caused by scabies and lice.
Olanzapine is an antipsychotic medication used to treat psychiatric disorders.
Phenergan is an antihistamine used to treat allergic reactions and alleviates pruritis.
Ondansetron is an antinausea medication used to help prevent and/or treat nausea and vomiting due to illness or induced by certain medications such as chemotherapy agents.

143. C: Calcium-rich foods help prevent gout flare-ups. Coffee and foods rich in vitamin C also help reduce a patient's risk. Patients should be counseled to refrain or severely limit their intake of red meat, seafood, alcohol, and fructose. Medications used to prevent gout include allopurinol, nonsteroidal anti-inflammatory drugs (NSAIDs), and steroids. Colchicine is most commonly used to treat acute gout attacks.

144. C: This patient has infective endocarditis caused by her drug use. Endocarditis causes a number of symptoms, but the most classic are fever, chills, and diaphoresis. Common causes are indwelling triple-lumen catheters or peripherally inserted central catheter (PICC) lines, dental procedures, and intravenous (IV) drug abuse with contaminated needles. Janeway lesions indicate a diagnosis of endocarditis. These lesions are painful, erythematous areas on the palms and soles, which are only caused by endocarditis.

145. D: Restrictive cardiomyopathy is the inability of the heart to relax between beats.
Epinephrine is a vasoconstrictor, which would increase the workload of a heart that is already impaired.
Furosemide and metoprolol decrease the heart rate as well as decrease the preload and afterload on the heart.
The blood is being squeezed through restricted vasculature, which increases the risk of developing clots. Aspirin helps prevent the formation of clots and is commonly used in the treatment of restrictive cardiomyopathy.

146. B: Toxic megacolon is a complication of *Clostridium difficile* colitis. It is the pathologic distension of the colon caused by *C. difficile*, Crohn's disease, and ulcerative colitis. Signs and symptoms may include tachycardia, abdominal pain, abdominal distension, leukocytosis, and fever. The treatment is to decompress the colon either by rectal tube or by surgical intervention.
Ogilvie's syndrome is a condition in which a patient presents with signs and symptoms of intestinal obstruction without actually having an obstruction. The bowel loses its ability to contract and to pass food and waste products along the gastrointestinal (GI) tract; this commonly occurs after surgery or in severely chronically ill patients.
Intussusception is when one part of the bowel folds in on itself and causes an obstruction. This is common in children. Symptoms include nausea, vomiting, lethargy, and "red currant jelly" stools.

Hirschsprung's disease is a congenital condition in which the bowel cannot contract and move food and waste products along the GI tract due to lack of nerve innervation of portions of the bowel.

147. C: This patient has alcohol-induced pancreatitis. Alcohol is the leading cause of acute pancreatitis; stones are the second most common cause. Therapies include cessation of alcohol, rest, intravenous (IV) fluids, pain medications, keeping the patient on nothing-by-mouth (NPO) status, and antibiotics in the presence of a secondary infection.
Hepatitis and cholangitis would present with right-sided abdominal pain, along with fever, chills, nausea, vomiting, and possibly jaundice.
Mallory–Weiss tears may be also caused by alcoholism, but they occur in the esophagus and do not cause abdominal pain.

148. C: This patient most likely has Parkinson's disease. The classic four signs of Parkinson's disease are resting tremor, rigidity, slow movements, and shuffling gait. It is due to the deterioration of the substantia nigra.
Guillain–Barré syndrome is an autoimmune disease causing muscle weakness or paralysis. It does not cause resting tremor or rigidity.
Huntington's disease is a progressive neurological disorder caused by an autosomal-dominant chromosomal abnormality. Signs include progressive decline in cognitive function; ataxic gait; and uncoordinated, jerky body movements.
Alzheimer's disease is the development of progressive cognitive decline; the underlying cause is not known. Motor skills are much less affected until late stages of the disease.

149. A: This patient has an excess of cortisol due to her exogenous steroid use, causing Cushing's syndrome. Cushing's syndrome symptoms include buffalo hump (posterior cervical fat pad), swelling of the face, myalgias, unintentional weight gain, irregular menses, striae, hirsutism, hyperglycemia, and bone loss.

150. B: This patient is most likely suffering from Stevens–Johnson syndrome caused by a reaction she's having to penicillin. It is a reaction of the skin and mucous membranes to medication or to a medical condition. It begins with nonspecific upper respiratory infection symptoms and then progresses to dermal manifestations. It can be life threatening if not treated immediately and adequately.
Cushing's syndrome is caused by too much cortisol, causing symptoms such as buffalo hump (posterior cervical fat pad), swelling of the face, myalgias, unintentional weight gain, irregular menses, striae, hirsutism, hyperglycemia, and bone loss.
Guillain–Barré syndrome is an autoimmune disease causing muscle weakness or paralysis.
Turner syndrome is a genetic condition in which females are missing all or part of an X chromosome. Some of the symptoms may include infertility, amenorrhea, short stature, and webbed neck.

151. A: The child most likely had idiopathic thrombocytopenic purpura (ITP) caused by his viral syndrome. It is characterized by petechiae or a pinpoint rash seen on the extremities. In children, ITP usually resolves on its own without treatment.
Stevens–Johnson syndrome begins with nonspecific upper respiratory infection symptoms and then progresses to dermal manifestations. The rash is a diffuse, dark red macular and papular rash with extensive blistering usually requiring hospitalization. It can be life threatening if not treated immediately and adequately.
Von Willebrand disease is a milder form of hemophilia. It is caused by factor VIII deficiency. Symptoms include prolonged bleeding after dental or surgical procedures, minor injuries, and menorrhagia.

Glucose-6-phosphate dehydrogenase (G6PD) deficiency is an X-linked recessive hereditary disease in which the defect of this enzyme causes red blood cells to break down prematurely. It causes pallor, dark urine, jaundice, and failure to thrive. It is generally diagnosed in infancy. Symptoms do not spontaneously resolve.

152. D: The child has diphtheria. It is a very rare respiratory infection in developed countries due to the diphtheria, tetanus, and pertussis (DTaP) vaccine, but children can still get diphtheria if they are not vaccinated. Signs and symptoms include a grayish-black, tough, fiberlike covering of the oropharynx, fever, chills, sore throat, cyanosis, and in severe cases drooling and stridor.
Cryptococcus infections are generally seen in patients who are immunocompromised. Cryptococcus is a fungus that people with normal immune systems can handle. There is no vaccine to prevent against cryptococcus infections.
Shigella causes bacterial gastroenteritis.
Cholera is a rare bacterial gastroenteritis that may cause severe dehydration and death.

153. D: The child has mononucleosis caused by the Epstein–Barr virus. Conservative treatment such as rest, fluids, and refraining from physical activity to prevent splenic rupture are recommended.
Amantadine is an antiviral medication used within one to two days after the onset of flu symptoms to help shorten the duration of the illness.
Augmentin would be used if the child had a bacterial upper respiratory infection.
A computed tomography (CT) scan of the abdomen is not recommended if splenic rupture is not suspected.

154. B: This patient has multiple myeloma, which is a type of cancer of the plasma cells. The most common signs and symptoms are bone pain and pathologic fractures. Multiple myeloma can also cause damage to the kidneys, causing anemia. The presence of the Bence Jones protein in the urine distinguishes this as the most likely diagnosis from Paget's disease, which can also cause bone pain and pathologic fractures.
Acute myelogenous leukemia (AML) is a cancer of the blood and bone marrow, usually presenting with bleeding, bruising, fatigue, and weight loss.
Acute lymphocytic leukemia (ALL) is a cancer of the white blood cells, usually presenting with weight loss, fatigue, petechiae, and fever.

155. A: The international normalized ratio (INR) is generally used to measure bleeding time. This lab test is important in monitoring a patient who is taking Coumadin or for the workup of a bleeding disorder. It is generally not used in the workup of hemolytic anemia.
The Coombs' test looks for antibodies that may attach themselves to red blood cells and cause premature apoptosis.
A complete blood count (CBC) may be able to indicate what type of anemia is present, whether the patient is pancytopenic, or if an underlying infection is present.
Lactate dehydrogenase (LDH) is present in blood cells; increased levels of LDH indicate hemolytic anemia.

156. A: Influenza is not responsible for causing the abnormalities seen in this infant. Microcephaly, deafness, chorioretinitis, hepatosplenomegaly, and thrombocytopenia are common signs and symptoms of TORCH infections. TORCH infections can be caused by toxoplasmosis, other (syphilis, varicella, human immunodeficiency virus [HIV]), rubella, cytomegalovirus, and herpes simplex virus – type 2 (HSV-2). Prognosis of the infant depends on which type of infection she has. Some TORCH infections can be prevented with vaccines, and others can be treated with antibiotics, but because most infections are viral, there is no cure.

157. C: Pasta, baked goods, and processed foods lack iron and therefore should be avoided or severely limited in patients who have iron-deficiency anemia. Meat, eggs, and beans are obviously rich in protein and iron, but green, leafy vegetables such as kale and spinach are also good sources of iron. Foods that have high vitamin C content such as oranges increase the body's ability to absorb iron.

158. D: This patient has lichen planus, which is commonly described as well-defined, pruritic, planar, purple, polygonal papules and plaques. It may occur on mucous membranes or on the skin. It is a benign condition. The exact cause is unknown. It is linked to some chronic diseases, such as hepatitis C. Leukoplakia is a condition in which white patches may develop on the tongue or inside the mouth. Impetigo is a bacterial infection that is most commonly caused by *Staphylococcus aureus* or *Streptococcus pyogenes*. It causes lesions that can occur anywhere on the body. The lesions are small, red, pus-filled and can crack open and form a yellow or honey-colored, thick crust. They occur most commonly in young children.
Psoriasis causes cells to build up rapidly on the surface of the skin, forming itchy, dry, red, raised patches covered with grayish silvery lesions that are easily friable. Psoriasis is sometimes painful. Plaques frequently occur on the skin of the elbows and knees, but they can affect any area. This is a chronic condition.

159. A: Dyshidrosis is a type of eczema most commonly linked to stress and allergies. It is characterized by pruritic blisters on the palms and soles. No antibiotics are warranted. Conservative measures such as the use of steroids, emollients, and Benadryl are used for symptomatic relief. It is recommended that patients not scratch their lesions because scratching may exacerbate symptoms and cause secondary infection. This is a chronic condition.

160. B: Lantus would be the first-line treatment in a patient with newly diagnosed diabetes mellitus – type 1. Type 1 diabetes is an autoimmune disease in which the body attacks the islets of Langerhans of the pancreas. The islets of Langerhans have beta cells, which produce insulin. Patients who are type 1 diabetics are insulin dependent their whole lives. Although other agents may be added later on to help control hyperglycemia, insulin is the first-choice drug.

161. C: The patient is suffering from acute alcohol withdrawal. He states that he has not had an alcoholic beverage in two days. Symptoms may start as soon as a few hours after the last drink or may take two to three days to appear. Signs and symptoms may include tachycardia, nausea, vomiting, diarrhea, diaphoresis, confusion, headaches, seizures, fine motor tremor, and dilated pupils.
The patient is confused, but he is not delusional.
Dysthymic disorder is a milder form of major depressive disorder.

162. D: The patient has Osgood–Schlatter disease, which is an inflammation of the anterior tibial tubercle due to overuse while the bone is still growing. It is most commonly seen in prepubescent boys. Pain medications may be used, and rest is recommended, but no intervention is warranted. Symptoms will resolve eventually.
An anterior cruciate ligament (ACL) disruption is not likely because there is no history of trauma and there is no joint laxity or instability on physical examination.
Polymyositis is the appearance of bilateral muscle weakness and wasting due to immune disorders or disease.
Ganglion cysts may develop due to trauma, overuse, or idiopathic causes. They most commonly appear on the hands and feet.

163. A: Prednisone is a common medication used to treat polyarteritis nodosa. Polyarteritis nodosa is a vasculitis that affects small and medium-sized arteries, causing a large range of nonspecific symptoms.

There is no known cause, but the incidence is higher in men than women, and people with hepatitis B have a higher incidence of developing this disorder. Treatment includes steroids and immunosuppressive drugs such as methotrexate.

Antibiotics such as clindamycin are not warranted.

Permethrin cream is an insecticide used to treat skin infections caused by scabies and lice.

Amantadine is a medication used to treat attention deficit-hyperactivity disorder (ADHD) and has been used to treat Parkinson's disease and influenza.

164. B: Condyloma acuminata, or genital warts, is a sexually transmitted disease. Factors such as birth control use, smoking, early age of first coitus, and multiple sexual partners increase the risk of contracting genital warts. There is no cure; however, there are gels and creams that help with the symptoms and the appearance of the warts. Cryosurgery and laser surgery may be useful for acute exacerbations, but warts may still come back after the procedure. The human papilloma virus (HPV) vaccine is available to help prevent genital warts.

165. D: Acromegaly will result in the presence of excessive growth hormone in an adult patient. Because adult patients have already stopped growing, growth hormone will cause bones to thicken and widen, causing pain, weakness, and deformity. If excessive growth hormone occurs in children, gigantism will occur because bones are still in the process of growing longitudinally.

Dwarfism occurs when there is a deficiency in growth hormone.

Cushing's syndrome occurs in the presence of excessive cortisol.

166. C: This patient most likely has multiple sclerosis (MS). One of the most common presenting symptoms is persistent fatigue. One of the most common signs is optic neuritis. Two-thirds of MS patients will experience optic neuritis during the course of their disease. Patients may also present with progressive ataxia, muscle spasms, dizziness, ataxia, uncoordination of fine motor movements, urinary frequency, incontinence, nystagmus, and depression.

Huntington's disease is a progressive neurological disorder caused by an autosomal-dominant chromosomal abnormality. Signs include progressive decline in cognitive function; ataxic gait; and uncoordinated, jerky body movements.

Alzheimer's disease is a progressive cognitive decline. The underlying cause is not known. Motor skills are much less affected until late stages of the disease.

Meningitis is an infection that classically presents with nuchal rigidity, photophobia, and headache.

167. B: This patient most likely has parotitis. The parotid gland is one of the salivary glands; when they get infected, a patient may display dry mouth, drooling, facial swelling, and pain inside of the cheek.

Sjögren's syndrome is an immune disorder in which mucous membranes and moisture-secreting glands produce insufficient tears and saliva. Patients with Sjögren's disease have an increased risk of parotitis.

A peritonsillar abscess is an infection of the tonsils; patients generally do not present with cheek pain. A patient may present with drooling, facial swelling, difficulty swallowing, sore throat, and dysphonia.

Leukoplakia is a condition in which white patches may develop on the tongue or inside the mouth. It is similar in appearance to oral thrush, except that in cases of thrush, the white lesions may be scraped off.

Epiglottitis commonly affects children, but it can occur in adults. It is an infection of the epiglottis. Patients will present with upper respiratory infection (URI) symptoms, drooling, dysphonia, stridor, and fever. Sometimes, a patient will hold his or her head forward with the neck extended to keep the airways open.

168. A: The patient has aphthous ulcers, which are non-life-threatening and do not require antibiotics or antiviral medication.

Nonsteroidal anti-inflammatory drugs (NSAIDs), nonalcoholic mouth wash, and steroids are most commonly used to prevent future sores and alleviate the symptoms of present sores. The cause of aphthous ulcers is unknown, but dietary deficiencies in iron and folic acid, trauma, and emotional stress are thought to be potential triggers.

169. B: If testicular torsion is suspected, a stat surgical consult is warranted because the only correction of torsion is surgery. Surgery should be performed within six hours of the trauma in order to save the testicle. If blood flow is compromised for too long, the testicle may need to be removed.
Pain medications should be given, but a surgical consult should be called first.
The patient may need preoperative antibiotics for prophylaxis, depending on the surgeon's preferences, but it should not be the next step in management because testicular torsion is not due to infection.
Warm compresses would help if the patient had an abscess or testicular swelling without torsion, but they would provide very little benefit in this scenario.

170. D: This patient most likely has diabetes insipidus caused by her traumatic head injury. Diabetes insipidus is caused by insufficient antidiuretic hormone (ADH), which causes the body to conserve little, if any, water. This condition may be caused by trauma, surgery, or infection. In this case, it is most likely caused by the patient's traumatic brain injury.
Diabetes mellitus occurs when the body's insulin production is insufficient to meet a patient's glucose intake. Patients with diabetes mellitus will have high glucose levels in their blood and urine; those with diabetes insipidus do not.
Hypothyroidism causes a slowing in metabolism and potentially impaired cognitive function, producing symptoms such as unintentional weight gain, low blood pressure, bradycardia, weakness, myxedema, and slow speech.
Hyperthyroidism causes an increase in metabolism, producing symptoms such as unintentional weight loss, high blood pressure, tremor, palpitations, and weakness.

171. C: This patient most likely has melanoma. The definitive way to make the diagnosis is via biopsy. The way to help diagnose melanoma on physical examination is to think of the mnemonic ABCDE: asymmetry, borders, color, diameter, and evolving over time. Melanoma frequently occurs as asymmetric lesions with irregular borders, with multiple colors within one lesion, with a diameter greater than 6 mm, and whose appearance changes or evolves over time.
Squamous-cell carcinoma is usually described as a light-colored, scaly crust on an erythematous base. It is usually found on sun-exposed areas.
Impetigo is a bacterial infection that is most commonly caused by *Staphylococcus aureus* or *Streptococcus pyogenes*. It causes lesions that can occur anywhere on the body. They are small, red, pus-filled and can crack open and form a yellow or honey-colored, thick crust. They occur most commonly in young children.
Basal-cell carcinoma is the most common type of skin cancer. It is usually described as a pearly pink or flesh-colored lesion that is easily friable and does not heal.

172. D: This patient most likely has bladder carcinoma. The definitive way to diagnose this man is through imaging of his abdomen and pelvis.
Wilms' tumor is a common renal tumor in pediatric patients. The exact cause is unknown, but the incidence does increase with family history, suggesting there is a genetic component. Symptoms may include abdominal pain, abdominal mass, nausea, vomiting, constipation, and changes in urine color. Hemihypertrophy and aniridia may be associated with this disease.
Prostatitis is an infection of the prostate gland, causing similar symptoms to that of a urinary tract infection (UTI). Although this patient does have some symptoms of a UTI, his unintentional weight loss and history of tobacco abuse point to carcinoma rather than infection.

Orchitis is an infection of the testicles, which can cause UTI symptoms, testicular pain and swelling, hematospermia, and painful intercourse.

173. A: A corneal abrasion is a scratch on the cornea of the eye, which causes a foreign-body sensation, pain, and conjunctival erythema. Patients should be prescribed an antibiotic such as erythromycin or gentamicin to prevent infection. Patients who wear contact lenses should also be advised to wear eyeglasses while they are on antibiotics so that their abrasion may heal without further complication. The other three medication choices listed are used to treat glaucoma.

174. C: Desmopressin is another name for antidiuretic hormone (ADH), which is used in treating those who have diabetes insipidus. Diabetes insipidus is caused by insufficient ADH, which causes the body to conserve little, if any, water.
Detrol is used in women who experience urinary urgency and frequency due to an overactive bladder.
Depakote is used to treat neurologic conditions such as seizures and migraines.
Decadron is a steroid used to treat certain types of skin disorders and autoimmune diseases.

175. A: The child is potentially being abused at home either by her mother or another person. When an examiner notices burns in a "glove and stocking" distribution, it usually means that the child's extremity is forcefully being placed into something hot and not that something was accidentally spilled. If an accidental spill occurs, you would see a much more irregular pattern, and it is usually only on one side of the extremity. Calling social services such as the Division of Youth and Family Services (DYFS) would be appropriate considering the appearance of the burns and the fact that this is the fourth occurrence.

176. C: Zofran is used to treat and prevent nausea and vomiting. It does not play a role in the medical management of schizophrenia.
Seroquel is a selective serotonin reuptake inhibitor (SRRI) used to treat anxiety, depression, and schizophrenia.
Haldol is a dopamine antagonist used to treat schizophrenia as well as other psychotic disorders.
Zyprexa is an antipsychotic medication used primarily to treat bipolar disorder and schizophrenia.

177. B: Actinic keratosis can appear as a flesh-toned, pink, gray, or reddish macule or papule with a scaly surface caused by overexposure to the sun. These lesions have a propensity for becoming squamous cell carcinomas, so it is recommended to patients to avoid prolonged sun exposure and to use sunscreen. They may be removed surgically if they cause cosmetic issues.

178. B: Paronychia is an abscess adjacent to the nail bed. This can occur on the fingers or the toes. The cause may be idiopathic, but there is usually a history of trauma or a break in the skin prior to the onset of symptoms. Treatment includes warm compresses, antibiotics, and sometimes incision and drainage of the wound.
Onychomycosis is a fungal infection of the nail, which causes the nail to thicken, become yellow or gray, and occasionally fall off.
Condyloma acuminata is the appearance of genital or anal warts due to a viral sexually transmitted disease.
Scabies is a skin infection usually occurring in the webs of the fingers and toes due to mites burrowing underneath the skin.

179. D: Vitiligo is the hypopigmentation of the skin that usually occurs symmetrically. It may occur in a localized area or in widespread areas on the body. It is more common in darker skinned people. This is a benign condition.
A lipoma is a benign tumor created by the overgrowth of fatty tissue.

- 83 -

Xanthelasma are raised, yellow patches on the eyelids. The incidence of occurrence increases with age. They are common in patients with hyperlipidemia.

Mongolian spots are flat, blue, or blue-gray skin markings near the buttocks that commonly appear at birth or shortly thereafter.

180. C: Morphine is a narcotic medication that can cause constipation. This medication would not be recommended in a patient with a history of fecal impaction because it may precipitate bowel motility issues.

Senna and Colace are stool softeners that may help make it easier to pass a bowel movement in a patient with a history of constipation.

Milk of Magnesia helps prevent water from being reabsorbed in the intestines. Because it increases the amount of water that remains in the bowels, it helps promote bowel movements.

181. D: Adenosine is a medication that is given to a patient experiencing supraventricular tachycardia. It is an antiarrhythmic agent used to slow down the heart rate. The first dose should be given as a 6 mg bolus. If unsuccessful, a 12 mg dose should follow in one to two minutes. The 12 mg may be repeated once if needed.

Atropine is a medication used to speed up the heart rate; it is given to patients experiencing symptomatic bradycardia.

Allopurinol is a medication given to patients to help prevent gout exacerbations.

Atorvastatin is a medication used to lower serum cholesterol levels.

182. A: Atropine, dopamine, and epinephrine are medications that can be given for a patient experiencing symptomatic bradycardia. The other choices given are antiarrhythmic agents, which are used to slow down a patient's heart rate.

Amiodarone may be given to patients having pulseless ventricular tachycardia/ventricular fibrillation or atrial fibrillation.

Vasopressin, like amiodarone, slows down the heart rate and is given in the presence of ventricular tachycardia or ventricular fibrillation.

Adenosine is given to a patient experiencing supraventricular tachycardia.

183. C: This patient is immune to hepatitis B due to prior vaccination. Hepatitis B surface antigen (HBsAg) is present in active or chronic infections. In this case, it is not present.

Total hepatitis B core antibody (anti-HBc) indicates previous or acute hepatitis B infection. In this case, it is not present.

Hepatitis B surface antibody (anti-HBs) is present is patients who are recovering from an infection or who have been immunized. Because the other two lab values are negative, this could only mean that the patient has been successfully vaccinated.

184. D: You should recommend that the patient see a vascular surgeon for a biopsy to confirm the diagnosis. You may start the patient on a course of low-dose steroids. Because patients with giant-cell arteritis are at risk for development of aneurysms and stroke, starting the patient on baby aspirin is recommended. Giant-cell arteritis is the inflammation of the blood vessels that supply blood flow to the head. Common symptoms include unilateral headache, burning or tingling on one side of the head, hearing loss, jaw pain, and hearing or vision changes.

Because there is no infection involved, starting antibiotics would not be helpful.

Giant-cell arteritis involves inflammation of the blood vessels, not malignancy of the blood vessels, so a referral to an oncologist would be of little value.

Monitoring the situation without starting medications or obtaining a biopsy is inappropriate management because patients with giant-cell arteritis are at risk for development of aneurysms and stroke.

185. B: This patient has hypothyroidism. Her thyroid-stimulating hormone (TSH) is attempting to stimulate the thyroid gland to make more thyroid hormone, but the thyroid is unable to produce sufficient thyroid hormone for the body. The pituitary recognizes that there is insufficient thyroid hormone circulating, so it produces more TSH in hopes of stimulating the thyroid more. The T3 levels may be normal or low normal in hypothyroidism because T4 is the active form of thyroid hormone made available to the body.

186. A: Oseltamivir, or Tamiflu, is an antiviral medication used to lessen the severity of flu symptoms if given early enough during the course of infection.
Acyclovir and famciclovir are also antiviral medications, but they are used primarily to treat acute herpes exacerbations. They may also be used in the treatment of herpes zoster.
Augmentin is an antibiotic used to treat bacterial upper respiratory infections. Because influenza is a viral infection, prescribing an antibiotic would be of little use.

187. C: This patient most likely has orthostatic hypotension, which is defined as a drop in systolic blood pressure by 20 mmHg and a drop of at least 10 mmHg in diastolic blood pressure when a patient moves from a supine to sitting position. Symptoms may include weakness, dizziness, headache, and syncope. Orthostatic hypotension may be caused by medications, or it may be due to prolonged bed rest, especially if it occurs in a hospital setting.

188. B: The patient is in hypertensive crisis. Hypertensive crisis is defined as a systolic blood pressure more than 180 and a diastolic blood pressure more than 120 with evidence of organ damage. The patient has proteinuria, which means that the kidneys are showing signs of damage.
Normal hypertension is defined as a systolic blood pressure less than 120 and a diastolic blood pressure less than 80.
Prehypertension is defined as a systolic blood pressure from 120 to 139 and a diastolic blood pressure from 80 to 89.
Stage 1 hypertension is defined as a systolic blood pressure from 140 to 159 and a diastolic blood pressure from 90 to 99.
Stage 2 hypertension is defined as a systolic blood pressure from 160 to 179 and a diastolic blood pressure of greater than 100.

189. D: The patient is displaying signs and symptoms of diabetes mellitus and needs further workup to confirm the diagnosis. Signs of diabetes include frequent hunger, frequent thirst, unintentional weight loss, numbness or paresthesias in the extremities, frequent urinary tract infections, and visual changes. The hemoglobin A1C (HA1C) test monitors the average serum glucose for the previous three months. If it is above 6.0, then the patient is diagnosed with diabetes. A complete blood count (CBC), basic metabolic panel, and urinalysis should be checked in a patient with suspected diabetes. If glucose is present in the urine, then patient has diabetes. A complete blood count (CBC) and basic metabolic panel (BMP) may show electrolyte abnormalities or show if there is a concurrent infection present.
The patient has a yeast infection, which should be treated with Diflucan; antibiotics won't treat a yeast infection. Pyridium helps alleviate dysuria, which is not one of the patient's symptoms.
Blood and urine cultures should be ordered if sepsis is suspected. The patient's vital signs are normal, so sepsis should not be a concern.

190. B: A varicocele is an enlargement of the veins in the scrotum, causing testicular aching and/or swelling to occur. The venous enlargement is usually due to faulty valves in the veins or compression of a neighboring vein disrupting blood flow in nearby veins. Palpation of the affected testicle is often described as feeling like "a bag of worms."

Testicular torsion is a medical emergency. It occurs when the spermatic cord becomes twisted and blood flow to the testicle is severely diminished or absent. It presents with acute onset of pain and swelling of the affected testicle.

Testicular carcinomas present as hard, painless, fixed testicular solid lesions.

A hydrocele is the collection of fluid around the testicle due to infection, malignancy, or unknown cause. It appears as a soft, usually painless mass on the testicle. They are not harmful and have no serious long-term complications.

191. A: Graves' disease is one of the most common causes of hyperthyroidism, causing tremor, unintentional weight loss, palpitations, goiter, hypertension, fatigue, nervousness, increased appetite, and exophthalmos.

Addison's disease is due to insufficient cortisol, causing nausea, vomiting, diarrhea, hypotension, and darkening of the skin color, making the patient look like he or she went tanning.

Cushing's disease is due to the presence of excessive cortisol, causing unintentional weight gain, striae, a fat pad or buffalo hump on the posterior neck, facial swelling, and fatigue.

Hashimoto's disease occurs when the immune system attacks the thyroid gland, causing hypothyroidism. Signs and symptoms of hypothyroidism include bradycardia, unintentional weight gain, puffy face, fatigue, muscle weakness, hair loss, and dry skin.

192. B: This patient is displaying symptoms most consistent with epididymitis. Epididymitis is commonly caused by *Escherichia coli*. In sexually active males, the causative organisms are likely gonorrhea (GC)/chlamydia.

Prostatitis and cystitis usually present with symptoms such as fever, chills, hematuria, dysuria, urgency, and frequency.

Pyelonephritis presents with nausea, vomiting, fever, shaking chills, anorexia, abdominal pain, and back pain. Symptoms are exacerbated when the patient is lying down because the kidneys are retroperitoneal organs.

193. C: Health-care workers or those who work in close contact with people who have tuberculosis would need to have 10 mm or greater induration to have a positive purified protein derivative (PPD) test.

A patient with a normal immune system, no underlying disease, is not a health-care worker, and doesn't have regular contact with tuberculosis (TB)-positive patients would need an induration of 15 mm to have a positive PPD test.

An induration of 2 mm in any patient is considered a negative test.

An induration of 5 mm or more is considered positive in any patient that is immunocompromised.

194. A: Graves' disease is one of the most common causes of hyperthyroidism, causing tremor, unintentional weight loss, palpitations, goiter, hypertension, fatigue, nervousness, increased appetite, and exophthalmos. Tests to confirm the diagnosis include a thyroid function panel and an ultrasound or computed tomography (CT) scan of the thyroid if a goiter is present.

195. A: This patient is in acute renal failure due to her lithium overdose. The patient is anuric, which means that the kidneys aren't working properly and are not able to remove the toxin from her blood. Dialysis will remove the toxin from her body so her kidneys can recover. Although the other choices are not necessarily incorrect, they are not the immediate courses of action needed to help treat this patient's renal failure.

196. C: Children younger than 6 months of age are not recommended to get the influenza vaccine. The vaccine is recommended for children 6 months to 18 years old. It is especially important for health-care

workers, immunocompromised individuals, people who are living in close quarters such as assisted living facilities and hospitalized patients, and pregnant women.

197. D: This patient most likely has Addison's disease. Addison's disease is due to insufficient cortisol produced by the adrenal glands, causing nausea, vomiting, diarrhea, hypotension, and darkening of the patient's skin color, making the person look like he or she went tanning. Due to the low cortisol levels, the patient will generally have low sodium levels, causing salty food cravings.

198. B: The patient has diabetes and should be advised to modify his diet and maintain an active lifestyle. A patient without diabetes should have an HA1C of less than 6.0. Because this patient's HA1C is 6.2, his body mass index (BMI) is normal, and he has no other past medical problems, his diabetes may be manageable with dietary modifications.
If his HA1C does not normalize in the next two to three months with dietary modifications, starting antihyperglycemic medications would be recommended.
His BMI is normal, so losing weight would not help.

199. D: Propecia is used to treat benign prostatic hypertrophy and baldness. Levitra, Cialis, and Viagra are all used to treat erectile dysfunction. These three medications increase the level of nitrous oxide, which allows for vasodilatation of the blood vessels. By increasing vasodilatation, the penis will stay erect longer and help reverse the symptoms of erectile dysfunction.

200. C: This patient has a negative purified protein derivative (PPD). No further intervention is required. A patient with a normal immune system, no underlying disease, is not a health-care worker, and doesn't have regular contact with tuberculosis (TB)-positive patients would need an induration of 15 mm to have a positive PPD test. Because the patient has no medical issues and works as a librarian, the size of her induration is considered to be a negative test result.
An induration of 2 mm in any patient is considered a negative PPD test result.
An induration of 5 mm or more is considered positive in any patient that is immunocompromised.
Health-care workers or those who work in close contact with people who have tuberculosis would need to have 10 mm or greater induration to have a positive PPD test.

201. C: In sexually active males, the causative organisms are likely to be gonorrhea (GC)/chlamydia. This patient most likely has been getting epididymitis due to GC/chlamydia from unprotected sex.
Epididymitis is also commonly caused by *E. coli*. If he did not have a history of having unprotected sex, *E. coli* would be the more likely causative organism, and a urology referral may be recommended.
Drinking plenty of fluids is general advice given to those who suffer from sickle-cell disease, nephrolithiasis, and those who get persistent urinary tract infections (UTIs). Fluid hydration would not help prevent epididymitis.
Avoiding red meat, alcohol, and seafood are recommendations generally given to those with gout or cardiovascular disease.

202. B: Diverticulosis is the presence of pockets in any organ or fluid-filled cavity. The potential for developing this condition increases with age. Development of these pockets does not cause symptoms. If an infection develops within the diverticula, then this condition is called diverticulitis.
Mallory–Weiss tears are usually found in the esophageal junction. They are commonly seen in alcoholic patients caused by persistent episodes of vomiting; however, any pathological process that causes forceful coughing or vomiting may cause a Mallory–Weiss tear.
Celiac sprue is an immune reaction that damages the lining of the small intestine and prevents it from absorbing important nutrients. It presents with nausea, vomiting, diarrhea, and abdominal pain, which occur after ingesting gluten products.

- 87 -

Intussusception is when one part of the bowel folds in on itself and causes an obstruction. This is common in children. Symptoms include nausea, vomiting, lethargy, and "red-currant-jelly" stools.

203. A: Colchicine is used for treatment of acute gout exacerbations. This medication would not be useful in treating septic arthritis. A patient with septic arthritis has an infection in the blood that is attacking a joint or joints. Obtaining blood cultures, lab work, getting a joint aspiration, and prescribing pain medications and intravenous (IV) antibiotics are several ways to help diagnose and treat this infection.

204. D: Celiac disease, or celiac sprue, is an immune reaction that damages the lining of the small intestine and prevents it from absorbing important nutrients. It presents as nausea, vomiting, diarrhea, and abdominal pain that occur after ingesting gluten products. The mainstay of treatment is to maintain a gluten-free diet to help prevent future exacerbations. If the disease is refractory to conservative management, patients may be prescribed corticosteroids.

205. A: This patient has a superficial venous thrombus (SVT), which is a blood clot in the leg below the popliteal vein. A blood clot in the popliteal vein or higher is referred to as a deep venous thrombus (DVT). DVTs have a 30% to 50% chance of migrating to the lung; this is called a pulmonary embolus, which carries a high mortality rate. Patients with SVTs have a much lower risk of complications and can be monitored as an outpatient without being placed on medications. Patients who are at high risk, such as those with cancer, sickle-cell disease, lower extremity trauma or surgery, women who are taking birth control pills, patients who are obese, or persons who are bedridden may be started on Coumadin or have an inferior vena cava (IVC) filter placed if Coumadin is contraindicated.

206. C: Nursemaid's elbow describes the dislocation of the elbow most commonly due to trauma. It most commonly occurs in children under the age of eight due to their hyperflexible joints and growing bones. Children usually have little to no pain and hold their affected extremity in a flexed and pronated position. A Greenstick fracture is most commonly seen in children due to the flexibility of their bones. It occurs when the bony cortex bends abnormally, causing a partial break.
A Lisfranc fracture is the fracture and dislocation of one or more of the metatarsals.
A Colles' fracture is a fracture and dorsal displacement of the distal radius. It is commonly referred to as a "dinner-fork deformity" on x-ray.

207. B: In vitro, the ductus arteriosus is a blood vessel in which blood travels from the heart to the lungs. It normally closes a few days after birth, but in patients in which it does not, it is called patent ductus arteriosus (PDA). A heart murmur may be auscultated. Tachypnea, poor feeding, failure to thrive, shortness of breath, and diaphoresis are signs and symptoms in those patients who have moderate-to-severe PDA. If the defect is small, the patient may not have any symptoms and can be monitored as an outpatient without medications.
Aspirin is generally avoided in children younger than age 16 because they have an increased risk of developing Reye's syndrome, which causes swelling of the liver and brain.
Indomethacin is the drug of choice used in patients with symptomatic PDA.
Surgical closure of this cardiac defect is generally reserved for those with large defects.

208. D: Ramipril is an antihypertensive medication and is not used in the treatment of benign prostatic hypertrophy. Proscar, Cardura, and Rapaflo are all medications used to treat benign prostatic hypertrophy. Alpha-blockers such as Cardura and Rapaflo help the muscle in the prostate to relax so it does not impinge on the urethra. Medications such as Proscar, which is a 5-alpha reductase inhibitor, help slow the growth of the prostate.

209. D: In a patient who displays strokelike symptoms, the first thing you should do is order a computed tomography (CT) scan of the brain without contrast. If the CT scan is negative, tissue plasminogen activator (tPA) may be started in this patient because he has no contraindications. Tissue plasminogen activator or a heparin infusion should never be started in a suspected stroke case without ordering a CT scan first; if the patient has a hemorrhagic stroke, these medications can exacerbate the bleed and potentially kill the patient. Although the patient's neurological examination should be continually reassessed, treatment should not be postponed.

210. A: *Clostridium difficile* (*C. difficile*) colitis is a common nosocomial (hospital-acquired) infection. It is caused by the alteration of one's normal gastrointestinal (GI) flora, usually caused by long-term antibiotic usage. Vancomycin by mouth is one of the treatments for *C. difficile* colitis. The other medication used is po Flagyl. Vancomycin IV cannot be used in the treatment of *C. difficile* because insufficient amounts of it reach the colon to have any effect. Azithromycin and clindamycin play no role in the treatment of *C. difficile* colitis. Clindamycin is one the antibiotics that runs an increased risk of causing *C. difficile* colitis.

211. C: Status epilepticus describes a patient who continuously seizes. Phenytoin is an antiseizure medication, and lorazepam is used for sedation; both medications are used to help treat status epilepticus. Levetiracetam is also used for the treatment of seizure disorders. Lomotil helps to treat diarrhea. Linezolid is an antibiotic. Neither Lomotil nor linezolid plays any role in the treatment of status epilepticus.

212. B: Virchow's triad includes hypercoagulability, endothelial injury, and hemodynamic changes that increase one's risk of thrombosis.
Charcot's triad is the combination of jaundice, fever, and right-upper quadrant abdominal pain. It occurs as a result of ascending cholangitis.
Cushing's triad is a clinical triad defined as hypertension, bradycardia, and irregular respirations. It suggests rising intracranial pressure due to intracranial pathology such as hemorrhage.
Beck's triad is the combination of distended jugular veins, hypotension, and muffled heart sounds. It occurs as a result of pericardial effusion.

213. B: This patient may have a Lisfranc fracture. A Lisfranc fracture is the fracture and dislocation of one or more of the metatarsals.
Monteggia's fracture is a fracture of the ulna and dislocation of the radius.
A Colles' fracture is a fracture and dorsal displacement of the distal radius. It is commonly referred to as a "dinner-fork deformity" on x-ray.
A Le Fort fracture is a fracture of the maxilla; this type of fracture has four categories based on the severity of the fracture.

214. B: Amiodarone is an antiarrhythmic medication used for diseases such as atrial fibrillation. It plays no role in the treatment of cystic fibrosis nor does it prevent complications that may be associated with cystic fibrosis.
Mucinex helps thin out the copious mucus that collects in the airways of those with cystic fibrosis. By thinning out the mucous, the patient is able to expectorate it more easily, which helps prevent infection. Albuterol is a bronchodilator that opens up the airways and makes it easier to breathe for those with pulmonary diseases such as cystic fibrosis, asthma, and chronic obstructive pulmonary disease (COPD). Nonsteroidal anti-inflammatory drugs (NSAIDs) such as Motrin help decrease inflammation, which can help with infections and prevent airway damage.

215. D: Pott's disease is caused by the spread of tuberculosis to the spine. Signs and symptoms may include night sweats, anorexia, back pain, and lower extremity weakness.

Parkinson's disease destroys dopamine-producing neurons in the substantia nigra, and it causes motor symptoms (dyskinesia, tremor, and rigidity) as well as cognitive symptoms.

Hashimoto's disease occurs when the immune system attacks the thyroid gland, causing hypothyroidism. Signs and symptoms of hypothyroidism include bradycardia, unintentional weight gain, puffy face, fatigue, muscle weakness, hair loss, and dry skin.

Cushing's disease is due to the presence of excessive cortisol, causing unintentional weight gain, striae, a fat pad or buffalo hump on the posterior neck, facial swelling, and fatigue.

216. A: Fibromyalgia is a diagnosis of exclusion. Patients often complain of generalized body aches and pains with no known cause found during a workup. It is linked to anxiety and depression in many cases.

Polyarteritis nodosa is a type of vasculitis with unknown cause. Signs and symptoms of this disease may include painful red bumps on the skin, myalgias, fever, arthralgias, and weakness. It is diagnosed through a variety of lab tests and a biopsy.

Osteoarthritis is the degeneration of one or more joints usually diagnosed by x ray.

Polymyalgia rheumatica is a type of rheumatoid disease, which usually affects the larger joints such as the shoulders and hips. It is diagnosed by a variety of lab tests, which show the presence of inflammation, as well as by physical examination.

217. D: Paroxetine is used to treat generalized anxiety disorder, depression, posttraumatic stress disorder, as well as other psychiatric conditions.

Prednisolone is a type of steroid used to treat inflammatory reactions, such as localized skin reactions and asthma.

Promethazine is used to treat and prevent nausea and vomiting. It is also used for motion sickness.

Permethrin is used to treat infections caused by scabies.

218. C: This patient has cataracts, which are sclerotic lesions on the lens that slowly obstruct vision. They become more common with age. Surgical intervention alleviates symptoms.

Conjunctivitis is an infection of the clear portion of the eye called the conjunctiva, which may present with conjunctival erythema, pain or discomfort, itching, discharge, and crusting of the lids or lashes.

A hyphema is a hemorrhage in the anterior portion of the eye, which can be due to inflammation or trauma. It may cause pain or visual disturbances.

Blepharitis is inflammation of the eyelids, causing them to become red and painful. This condition is caused by localized trauma or irritation.

219. B: Doppler ultrasound is the treatment of choice in diagnosing deep venous thromboses. It is very sensitive and exposes the patient to the least amount of radiation.

Computed tomography (CT) and magnetic resonance imaging (MRI) scans are usually reserved for tissue, muscular, or ligamentous injuries or pathologies. They are also good in diagnosing infections or fluid collections.

X rays are not used because they only show bones. They do not show muscles, ligaments, tissues, or blood vessels.

220. A: Mallory–Weiss tears occur in the esophageal junction and are usually seen in alcoholic patients caused by persistent episodes of vomiting. However, any pathological process that causes forceful coughing or vomiting may cause a Mallory–Weiss tear.

In Crohn's disease, the colon wall may have a "cobblestone" appearance due to the intermittent pattern of affected and nonaffected colonic tissue.

Ulcerative colitis usually affects continuous stretches of the colon and rectum.

Whipple's disease is a rare, chronic disease caused by bacterial infection. The affected bowel is usually swollen with raised, yellowish patches.

221. D: This patient most likely has a venous thrombus caused by her recent hip surgery. Patients with venous thromboses have a positive Homan's sign in approximately one-third of the cases. A positive Homan's sign may be elicited if a patient has pain with dorsiflexion of his or her foot while the leg is extended.

Osteomyelitis and septic arthritis are unlikely because they are involved with infection of a joint or joints rather than presenting with muscular pain and swelling.

Osgood–Schlatter disease is the swelling of the tibial tubercle, which commonly occurs in pubescent and prepubescent children.

222. A: Mitral regurgitation is occurring on the two-dimensional echocardiography (2D echo). The mitral valve permits blood flow from the left atrium into the left ventricle. If the valve does not close properly, mitral regurgitation will occur.

Pulmonic regurgitation is the backflow of blood from the pulmonary artery into the right ventricle.

Tricuspid regurgitation is the backflow of blood from the right ventricle into the right atrium.

Aortic regurgitation is the backflow of blood from the aorta into the left ventricle.

223. C: You would give 1 mg of epinephrine, or you could give 40 units of vasopressin. Because vasopressin is not an option, epinephrine would be the drug of choice, according to Advanced Cardiovascular Life Support (ACLS) protocol. Amiodarone, lidocaine, and magnesium sulfate could be given during a code involving a patient with pulseless ventricular tachycardia, but they would be given after the administration of vasopressin or epinephrine.

224. B: This patient most likely has gynecomastia, which is the appearance of breasts in males due to enlarged mammary glands. This may due to obesity, congenital etiology, endocrine abnormality, or underlying disease. This condition usually resolves on its own in a patient with no significant past medical history.

Fibroadenomas are generally singular, rubbery, nontender breast lesions that are benign in nature.

Malignant breast masses are generally nontender breast lesions and usually do not occur bilaterally.

Fibrocystic breast disease is a benign condition in which singular or multiple breast cysts develop. They can occur right before one's menses begins, or they may be unrelated to menses. People placed on hormone replacement therapy or birth control pills generally have less severe symptoms.

225. A: The child has otitis media, which is an infection of the inner ear.

Mastoiditis is an infection of the mastoid bone of the skull. It is generally a complication of inner ear infections. Symptoms may include fever, ear pain, ear discharge, swelling behind the ear (where the mastoid bone is located), hearing loss, headache, and erythema. Imaging studies such as magnetic resonance imaging (MRI) and computed tomography (CT) scans can make a definitive diagnosis.

Acoustic neuromas are tumors of the acoustic nerve. They are much more common in adults than in children. Symptoms include hearing loss, dizziness, headache, tinnitus, facial droop, and ataxia.

Otitis externa is an infection of the outer ear. Signs and symptoms may include pain with palpation of the tragus, otorrhea, fever, and ear tugging.

226. B: This patient has meningitis. Meningitis is an infection that classically presents with nuchal rigidity, photophobia, and headache. The patient has a history of human immunodeficiency virus (HIV); being immunocompromised can predispose a person to developing meningitis. Kerning's sign is positive when a patient is unable to extend his or her leg when the hip is flexed. This maneuver helps diagnose meningitis. Huntington's disease is a slow, progressive neurological disorder caused by an autosomal-dominant chromosomal abnormality. Signs include progressive decline in cognitive function; ataxic gait; and uncoordinated, jerky body movements.

Schistosomiasis is a chronic parasitic infection due to eating improperly cooked pork. On magnetic resonance imaging (MRI) or computed tomography (CT) scan of the brain, it can appear as multiple enhancing nodules occurring in bilateral cerebral hemispheres.

Guillain–Barré syndrome is an autoimmune disorder in which the body attacks its own nervous system. The cause is generally unknown, but being immunocompromised or getting over a viral infection such as mononucleosis increases the risk of developing this disorder. Signs and symptoms may include numbness, weakness, paresthesias of the extremities, ataxia, dysphagia, and muscle spasms.

227. B: This patient most likely has bacterial meningitis. Neutrophil counts are elevated in patients with bacterial meningitis. Their glucose levels are low because bacteria use glucose. The level of protein in the spinal fluid goes up due to an increase in the presence of bacteria, which have a high composition of protein. Also, there is an increase in the presence of cells that fight infection, which are also composed of protein. When bacteria destroy the body's cells (or vice versa), the protein is released, causing protein levels to rise.

In viral meningitis, the neutrophil count may be elevated, but usually lymphocytes are the predominant cells. The glucose level is normal because viruses do not use glucose. The protein level is near normal because viruses do not have a high composition of protein. The white blood cell (WBC) count may be normal or elevated.

Myasthenia gravis is an autoimmune disorder in which the body attacks the voluntary muscles, causing facial droop or asymmetry, ataxia, muscle spasms, dysphagia, and airway difficulties. A lumbar puncture would be normal in a patient with myasthenia gravis.

Huntington's disease is a slow, progressive neurological disorder caused by an autosomal-dominant chromosomal abnormality. Signs include progressive decline in cognitive function; ataxic gait; and uncoordinated, jerky body movements. A lumbar puncture would be normal.

228. D: This patient has a respiratory acidosis. The pH is low (normal value 7.35 to 7.45), and the $PaCO_2$ is high (normal value 35 to 45). To interpret an arterial blood gas, first look at the pH. If it is low, acidosis is present. If the pH is high, alkalosis is present.

Next look at the $PaCO_2$; if it is low, alkalosis is present. If it is increased, acidosis is present. If the $PaCO_2$ explains the change of pH, then it is respiratory disorder. If it does not, look at the $HCO_3$. The normal range is 22 to 26. If the $HCO_3$ is increased and the pH is high, then you have metabolic alkalosis. If the pH is low and the $HCO_3$ is low, then you have metabolic acidosis.

229. C: This patient has normal pressure hydrocephalus (NPH). The common triad seen with NPH patients is ataxia, urinary incontinence, and dementia. The opening pressure of a lumbar puncture is normal (hence, "normal pressure" hydrocephalus). The ventricles, however, are enlarged on computed tomography (CT) or magnetic resonance imaging (MRI) scan. The treatment is to perform a lumbar puncture to determine if the symptoms resolve or improve. If they do, then the patient will most likely need a ventricular peritoneal shunt (VPS). NPH can occur without a cause, or it may be due to trauma such an aneurysm rupture, infection, or postsurgical complication.

A hygroma is a collection of cerebrospinal fluid in the subdural space. Acute hygromas are usually caused by head trauma or recent neurosurgical procedure.

Medulloblastomas are the most common malignant brain tumor and are significantly more common in children than in adults. They usually occur in the cerebellum.

An intraventricular hemorrhage is the presence of blood within the ventricles, most commonly due to hypertension. On this patient's CT scan, hydrocephalus, not blood, was noted.

230. A: This patient has anorexia nervosa. It is an eating disorder much more common in girls than boys, and it is most common in adolescents. It is characterized by purposely starving oneself in order to lose weight.

Bulimia nervosa is an eating disorder much more common in girls than boys and most common in adolescents. It involves periods of bingeing followed by periods of fasting in order to lose weight.

Generalized anxiety disorder is a psychiatric disorder in which a person feels anxious or nervous most or all of the time with no known cause.

Bipolar disorder is a psychiatric disorder in which a person has episodes of mania, or extreme happiness and energy, followed by periods of depression.

231. B: This patient has generalized anxiety disorder. Generalized anxiety disorder is a psychiatric disorder in which a person feels anxious or nervous most or all of the time with no known cause. Posttraumatic stress disorder (PTSD) is when a person feels nervous or anxious all or most of the time due to a known cause, such as the death of a loved one, rape, near-death experience or being involved in a disturbing event such as a school shooting or terrorist attack.

A phobia is feeling extremely nervous or scared about a particular stimulus that is usually nonthreatening to most people (i.e., being afraid to go outside or being afraid of water).

Dysthymic disorder is a milder form of major depressive disorder.

232. C: This patient has metabolic alkalosis. The pH is high, the $PaCO_2$ is normal, and the $HCO_3$ is high. To interpret an arterial blood gas, first look at the pH. If it is low, acidosis is present. If the pH is high, alkalosis is present. Next look at $PaCO_2$; if it is low, acidosis is present. If it is increased, alkalosis is present. If the $PaCO_2$ explains the change of pH, then it is respiratory disorder. If not, look at the $HCO_3$. The normal range is 22 to 26. If the $HCO_3$ is increased and the pH is high, then it indicates metabolic alkalosis. If the pH is low and the $HCO_3$ is low, it is metabolic acidosis.

233. C: This patient has normal pressure hydrocephalus (NPH) and should undergo a ventricular peritoneal shunt (VPS) if he or she is not a high-risk patient. There is no other way to correct NPH. Performing an electroencephalogram (EEG) may help rule out other etiologies that are causing the patient's symptoms, but it is not a treatment of NPH.

A magnetic resonance image (MRI) scan of the brain may help diagnose NPH and reveal its cause, but it is not a treatment of NPH.

A repeat lumbar puncture is not useful. Once a patient has one lumbar puncture and his or her symptoms improve, the diagnosis is made.

234. D: This patient has a phobia disorder; she has anthropophobia, which is a fear of people. A phobia is feeling extremely nervous or scared about a particular stimulus that is usually nonthreatening to most people (i.e., being afraid to go outside or being afraid of water).

Generalized anxiety disorder is a psychiatric disorder in which a person feels anxious or nervous most or all of the time with no known cause.

Posttraumatic stress disorder (PTSD) is when a person feels nervous or anxious all or most of the time due to a known cause such as the death of a loved one, rape, or near-death experience or being involved in a disturbing event such as a school shooting or terrorist attack.

Dysthymic disorder is a milder form of major depressive disorder.

235. A: Genetic mutations are the most common cause of hypertrophic cardiomyopathy. Hypertrophic cardiomyopathy is an abnormal thickening of the cardiac fibers. The thickening of these fibers impairs the heart from filling with blood and its ability to pump out blood to the rest of the body. This condition is diagnosed by an echocardiogram. Surgery, implantation of a pacemaker, and medications may help alleviate the complications this condition may cause.

236. B: Chorea is not a minor manifestation of acute rheumatic fever according to the Jones criteria. **Major manifestations of acute rheumatic fever include the following:**

Erythema marginatum: raised, nonpruritic, pink rings on the trunk and inner surfaces of the limbs
Carditis: inflammation of the heart muscle
Chorea: rapid, uncontrolled body movements
Subcutaneous nodules: painless, firm collections of collagen fibers over bones or tendons
Polyarthritis: temporary migrating inflammation of the large joints

**Minor manifestations of acute rheumatic fever include the following:**
1) Fever (101 °F to 102 °F)
2) Arthralgia: joint pain without swelling
3) Elevated erythrocyte sedimentation rate (ESR) or C-reactive protein (CRP)
4) Leukocytosis
5) Prior episode of rheumatic heart disease
6) Heart block seen on an electrocardiogram (EKG)

237. D: Tricuspid regurgitation is the backflow of blood from the right ventricle into the right atrium.
Aortic regurgitation is the backflow of blood from the aorta into the left ventricle.
The mitral valve permits blood flow from the left atrium into the left ventricle. If the valve does not close properly, mitral regurgitation will occur.
Pulmonic regurgitation is the backflow of blood from the pulmonary artery into the right ventricle.

238. D: Atropine, epinephrine, dopamine, and transcutaneous pacing are used for patients with symptomatic bradycardia.
Atropine is used to increase the heart rate; in ventricular fibrillation, the heart rate is already abnormally fast, so atropine would only exacerbate this arrhythmia.
Vasopressin, epinephrine, lidocaine, magnesium sulfate, and amiodarone are all medications that may be used in pulseless ventricular fibrillation or pulseless ventricular tachycardia.

239. B: This patient has a respiratory alkalosis. To interpret an arterial blood gas, first look at the pH. If it is low, acidosis is present. If the pH is high, alkalosis is present.
Next look at $PaCO_2$; if it is low, alkalosis is present. If it is increased, acidosis is present. If the $PaCO_2$ explains the change of pH, then it is respiratory disorder. If it does not, look at the $HCO_3$. The normal range is 22 to 26. If the $HCO_3$ is increased and the pH is high, then it indicates metabolic alkalosis. If the pH is low and the $HCO_3$ is low, it is metabolic acidosis.

240. B: The patient has horizontal nystagmus, which is common after acute drug or alcohol intoxication. It is an involuntary, oscillating eye movement that occurs bilaterally and resolves once the toxins are out of the body.
Entropion is the inward turning of the upper or lower lid toward the eye.
Exotropia is a condition in which one eye is normal and the other eye deviates laterally.
Conjunctivitis is the infection of the cornea causing pain, blurry vision, conjunctival erythema, and crusting of the lids and/or lashes.

241. B: This patient has right bundle branch block. This conduction arrhythmia has a widened QRS complex and two R waves best seen in V1.
Atrial fibrillation is a type of tachycardia with irregularly irregular QRS complexes and no P waves.
Sinus tachycardia is defined as a heart rate greater than 100 beats per minute with regular QRS complexes preceded by P waves.
Torsades de pointes means "twisting of the points" around the isoelectric baseline of an electrocardiogram (EKG), which describes this polymorphic ventricular tachycardia.

242. A: This patient had a ministroke, or transient ischemic attack (TIA). A TIA is a temporary lack of or insufficient blood flow to the brain, causing strokelike symptoms that resolve on their own once the blood flow is restored. There is no permanent brain damage and no acute findings on radiological studies. A cerebral vascular accident (CVA) is a stroke. A CVA occurs when there is prolonged lack of or insufficient blood flow to a part of the brain leading to brain cell death, or infarction. There is no way to revive dead blood cells. Complications of a stroke depend on the size of and the location of the infarct. Complications may range from minimal neurological deficits (if any) to significant neurological deficits, or death.

243. C: Although all medical professionals are bound by the Health Insurance Portability and Accountability Act (HIPAA), which ensures patient privacy, there are instances in which a medical professional may share a patient's information. If a patient threatens to injure themselves or others, a medical professional may reach out to local authorities or family members to warn them of the patient's potential plans in order to ensure the safety of the patient and others.

244. A: The patient has entropion, or the inward turning of the lid toward the eye. This may cause excessive tearing or irritation of the eye; if it is severe enough, the patient may develop a corneal abrasion.
Ectropion is the outward turning of the lid away from the eye.
Exotropia is the lateral deviation of the eye.
Esotropia is the inward deviation of the eye.

245. D: This patient has oppositional-defiant disorder (ODD), which is an emotional and psychiatric disorder that causes patients to have labile moods and have problems getting along with and listening to others. There is no one cause; sometimes it runs in families, sometimes it is seen in children of parents who abuse alcohol or drugs, and sometimes it is seen in children whose parents have psychiatric disorders. In some cases, there is no known cause.
Adjustment disorder is when a patient has a problem adjusting to or getting used to new life events or circumstances.
Dysthymic disorder is a milder form of major depressive disorder.
Attention-deficit hyperactivity disorder is when a patient has high level of energy and a short attention span.

246. A: Colchicine is used for the treatment of acute gout.
Phlebitis is the presence of a superficial clot in an extremity (most commonly in the leg), which can cause pain, swelling, and erythema. Patients may be given antibiotics if a secondary infection is present. They may be given anticoagulation medications depending on their risk factors and past medical history. Typically, phlebitis can be treated on an outpatient basis, using analgesics such as nonsteroidal anti-inflammatory drugs (NSAIDs), warm compresses, and compression stockings.

247. C: This patient has atrial fibrillation, which is a type of tachycardia with irregularly irregular QRS complexes and no P waves.
Sinus bradycardia is a heart rate less of than 60 beats per minute. It has regular QRS complexes preceded by P waves.
Right bundle branch block has a widened QRS complex and two R waves best seen in lead V1.
Sinus tachycardia is defined as a heart rate of greater than 100 beats per minute with regular QRS complexes preceded by P waves.

248. B: Frovatriptan is a tryptamine-based medication that helps prevent and treat migraine headaches. Other medications that may be used to treat migraines include nonsteroidal anti-inflammatory drugs (NSAIDs), aspirin, narcotics, and beta-blockers.

Fluoxetine is used to treat anxiety and depression.

Fexofenadine is an antihistamine used to treat seasonal allergy exacerbations.

Fluvastatin is part of the statin drug class that is used to treat hyperlipidemia.


249. D: A lumbar puncture may help aid in the diagnosis of this syndrome, but it is not used as a therapeutic aid, a preventative aid, or as a way to speed up recovery.

Guillain–Barré syndrome is an autoimmune disorder in which the body attacks its own nervous system. The cause is generally unknown, but being immunocompromised or getting over a viral infection such as mononucleosis increases the risk of developing this disorder. Signs and symptoms may include numbness and weakness of the extremities, respiratory distress, paresthesias of the extremities, ataxia, dysphagia, and muscle spasms.

Intubation is used in cases of respiratory distress to help maintain an open airway. Plasmapheresis and immunoglobulin therapy are methods used to help speed recovery.


250. B: Tourette disorder is first noticed in childhood and is characterized by involuntary verbal sounds and/or motor movements. It does not cause cognitive impairment, although it may be seen in the presence of cognitive disorders.

Alzheimer's disease is a progressive cognitive decline; the underlying cause is not known. Motor skills are much less affected until late stages of the disease.

Multiple sclerosis is a demyelinating disease, which may present with progressive ataxia, muscle spasms, dizziness, trouble with coordination of fine motor movements, urinary frequency, incontinence, nystagmus, and depression.

Huntington's disease is a progressive neurological disorder caused by an autosomal-dominant chromosomal abnormality, which usually occurs in the third or fourth decade of life. Signs include progressive decline in cognitive function; ataxic gait; and uncoordinated, jerky body movements.


251. A: Spirometry is the best test to aid in the diagnosis of chronic obstructive pulmonary disease (COPD). Spirometry measures airflow by testing lung volume and lung capacity.

A chest x ray may show pathological changes that accompany COPD, but the x ray may be normal. It is not a diagnostic test for COPD.

Auscultation with a stethoscope may reveal diminished breath sounds, but they can occur with many different conditions. Breath sounds may even be normal in someone with COPD.

An electrocardiogram (EKG) is the least helpful diagnostic aid; it generally is used to help diagnose cardiac-related abnormalities.


252. C: The sweat chloride test is the standard diagnostic test for cystic fibrosis.

A physical examination and past medical history of both the child and the parents are also important in making the diagnosis.

A chest x ray or a computed tomography (CT) scan of the chest may reveal pathologies such as pleural effusions, pneumonia, or bronchiectasis, but it is not diagnostic for cystic fibrosis.

A fecal fat test may help diagnose cystic fibrosis because complications with digestive fluids and pancreatitis are common in this patient population; however, there are other disease states in which a fecal fat test may be abnormal.


253. D: Aspergillosis is a fungal pneumonia commonly occurring in those who are immunocompromised. The classic radiological finding is a fungus ball seen on chest x ray or a computed tomography (CT) scan of the chest.

Sarcoidosis is a disease with an unknown cause in which granulomas can form in the organs or the skin. It is not a fungal disease.

Cystic fibrosis is an autosomal-recessive lung disorder in which mucus in the lungs and digestive tract becomes abnormally thick, causing chronic lung infections and gastrointestinal (GI) complications.

Pneumoconiosis, or "miner's lung," is a lung disease caused by long-term exposure to coal or coal-related products. A fungus ball is not seen on chest x ray because this is not a fungal disease.

254. C: Autism is a neurodevelopmental disorder affecting cognition and social skills. Signs may appear as early as a few weeks of life to as late as two or three years of age. Classic signs of this disorder are cognitive and social impairment and persistent repetitive behaviors. There is no known cause or cure. Speech therapy, behavioral therapies, psychiatric medications, and special education programs are the mainstays of treatment.

Adjustment disorder is when a patient has a problem getting used to new life events or circumstances.

Oppositional-defiant disorder (ODD) is an emotional and psychiatric disorder causing patients to have labile moods and have problems getting along with and listening to others. There is no one cause; sometimes it runs in families, sometimes it is seen in children of parents who abuse alcohol or drugs, and sometimes it is seen in children whose parents have psychiatric disorders. In some cases, there is no known cause.

Attention-deficit hyperactivity disorder is when a patient has high level of energy and a short attention span.

255. C: No intervention is needed if both the mother and baby are Rh-positive. The Rh factor is an antigen that may or may not be attached to one's blood cells. People with a positive blood type (A+, B+, O+, AB+) have the antigen. People with a negative blood type do not have the antigen and are Rh negative. If a mother is Rh negative and a child is Rh positive, RhoGAM needs to be administered. RhoGAM is an injection that suppresses the mother's immune response to the Rh-positive baby, which can help prevent hemolytic disease of the newborn or miscarriage.

Antibiotics are unnecessary because it is a blood incompatibility not an infection.

An ultrasound would be ineffective regarding Rh factor.

256. C: You should advise the patient that labor should be induced immediately. Eclampsia is the development of hypertension, proteinuria, and seizures during the second or third trimester. If the patient is at least 32 weeks pregnant, then she should be induced. The only cure for eclampsia is delivery. If the patient is less than 32 weeks pregnant, she may be managed on anticonvulsants and placed on a telemetry monitor for observation.

Blood transfusions play no role in the treatment or cure of eclampsia if the complete blood count is normal.

257. A: This patient has a pleural effusion, which is a pathologic fluid collection due to his chronic obstructive pulmonary disease (COPD). If the effusion is large enough, it will present with blunting of the costophrenic angle on chest x ray.

Aspergillosis is a fungal pneumonia commonly occurring in those who are immunocompromised. The classic radiological finding is a fungus ball seen on chest x ray or a computed tomography (CT) scan of the chest.

Pneumoconiosis, or "miner's lung," is a lung disease caused by long-term exposure to coal or coal-related products. The classic chest x-ray findings are small cystic radiolucencies that look like honeycombs on chest x ray.

Pneumothoraces will appear as a black space on a chest x ray with no lung markings. If they are small enough, the chest x ray may be normal.

258. D: A moderate-sized pneumothorax (typically one that is larger than 10% in size) will appear as a black space on chest x ray with no lung markings. If it is small (typically less than 10%), the chest x-ray may be normal.

Sarcoidosis is a disease with an unknown cause in which granulomas can form in one's organs or the skin. Pneumoconiosis, or "miner's lung," is a lung disease caused by long-term exposure to coal or coal-related products. The classic chest x-ray findings are small cystic radiolucencies that look like honeycombs on chest x ray.

259. A: Graves' disease is an autoimmune disease that causes hyperthyroidism, which would promote weight loss, not weight gain.

Untreated hypothyroidism may contribute to obesity because the thyroid plays a role in metabolism. If the thyroid is functioning more sluggishly than normal, weight gain may occur due to the slowing down of metabolism.

Cushing's disease is due to the presence of excessive cortisol, causing unintentional weight gain, striae, a fat pad or buffalo hump on the posterior neck, and facial swelling.

Women going through menopause are at an increased risk for gaining weight due to the various hormonal changes they are going through as well as a redistribution of body fat that commonly occurs during this time.

260. C: Allergic rhinitis is caused by a sensitivity or allergy to something in the environment. It is not a bacterial infection. Antibiotics are not prescribed for allergic rhinitis unless there is a secondary infection present.

Corticosteroids help treat inflammation commonly caused by an overactive immune system as well as help reduce swelling.

Decongestants help reduce the amount of fluid and mucus that accumulate in the airways.

Antihistamines are used to alleviate inflammation and pruritis.

261. D: Phobia disorder is a specific type of anxiety disorder. Although general anxiety disorder may not have a particular trigger or reason for the onset of symptoms, phobias are caused by a particular person, place, or thing. A phobia is feeling extremely nervous or scared about a particular stimulus that is usually nonthreatening to most people (i.e., being afraid to go outside or being afraid of water).

Ritalin is a psychostimulant used to help increase attention span and concentration; it is commonly used in patients who suffer from attention-deficit and hyperactivity disorder. It does not play a role in someone who suffers from phobias.

Xanax is a benzodiazepine, which will cause mild sedation. It is commonly used in those with schizophrenia, anxiety, and depression.

Metoprolol helps to lower blood pressure and heart rate. It is most commonly used in the treatment of hypertension and cardiac arrhythmias, but it may also be used in patients who suffer from phobias and stage fright.

Lexapro is a selective serotonin reuptake inhibitor (SSRI) used in the treatment of anxiety and depression.

262. B: Naloxone (Narcan) is an opiate antidote used to treat potential or confirmed narcotic overdoses. It is not used in the treatment of alcohol withdrawal.

There is no one treatment for alcohol withdrawal. Treatment is based on the symptoms displayed by the patient. Thiamine, magnesium, and folic acid are frequently administered to alcoholic patients because they are usually chronically malnourished and suffer from electrolyte imbalances due to their addiction.

Zofran is an antiemetic medication that prevents and alleviates nausea and vomiting.

Ativan is a benzodiazepine that causes mild sedation. It is usually given to alleviate symptoms such as delirium tremens.

263. C: This patient has a type of peritonsillar abscess called Ludwig's angina. It involves a bacterial infection under the tongue, causing swelling, erythema, dysphonia, dysphagia, and fever. The classic physical finding is a patient who sounds like he or she has a "hot potato in his or her mouth." It may occur spontaneously, but it is commonly preceded by a dental infection.

Acute pharyngitis is an infection of the pharynx that may cause dysphagia, dysphonia, and fever, but it does not commonly cause neck swelling and erythema and does not cause displacement of the tongue.

Aphthous ulcers are open sores that occur on the lips, gums, or tongue. The cause is unknown. They appear as gray, white, or yellow sores on an erythematous base. They may cause dysphagia, but they do not cause dysphonia, fever, neck swelling, or tongue displacement.

Oral leukoplakia is the presence of white plaques in the mouth caused by chronic irritation such as by chewing tobacco or from chronic disease. It does not cause dysphagia, dysphonia, tongue displacement, neck swelling, or erythema.

264. A: Irrigation of the eye would be generally ineffective and is not used in the treatment of a blowout fracture. A blowout fracture is a fracture of the walls and/or floor of the orbital bone most commonly caused by trauma.

Antibiotics are always warranted as prophylaxis against infection.

Steroids are used to help decrease swelling.

Surgery may be warranted depending on the severity of the fracture.

265. D: A Le Fort fracture is a fracture of the maxilla; this type of fracture has four categories based on severity.

A boxer's fracture is a transverse fracture of the fourth and/or fifth metacarpal bones usually as a result of trauma with a closed fist.

A Lisfranc fracture is the fracture and dislocation of one or more of the metatarsals.

A Colles' fracture is a fracture and dorsal displacement of the distal radius. It is commonly referred to as a "dinner-fork deformity" on x-ray.

266. D: The number-one cause of pelvic inflammatory disease (PID) is venereal disease, most notably, gonorrhea and chlamydia. Untreated sexually transmitted diseases may lead to PID, which is the primary preventable cause of infertility.

Approximately 10% to 15% of PID cases are caused by illnesses such as appendicitis or pelvic procedures such as dilation and curettage, abortion, or childbirth.

PID may be caused by a pelvic procedure, such as the removal of an ectopic pregnancy, or PID may cause an ectopic pregnancy to occur.

267. D: Esomeprazole is a proton pump inhibitor that causes the stomach to produce less acid. The reduction of acid production means that less acid is released into the esophagus, which will alleviate or partially alleviate symptoms and the damage done to the esophageal mucosa.

Metronidazole is an antibiotic used in treating anaerobic bacterial infections; it is also an amebicide and antiprotozoal medication.

Ketoconazole and fluconazole are antifungal medications.

268. A: A diverticulum is an outpouching of an organ or fluid-filled cavity. Meckel's diverticulum is two times more prevalent in boys than in girls. Meckel's diverticulum is usually two inches long and found approximately two feet from the ileocecal valve. Two years of age is the most common presentation for those with a complication involving Meckel's diverticulum. Approximately 2% of the population has this condition, although the majority of patients are asymptomatic.

269. B: Zollinger–Ellison syndrome is caused by tumors in the small intestine and pancreas that secrete gastrin, which can cause gastroesophageal reflux disease (GERD)-like symptoms, abdominal pain, hematemesis, and diarrhea.

Celiac sprue is an immune reaction that damages the lining of the small intestine and prevents it from absorbing important nutrients. A diagnosis can be made by an upper endoscopy with biopsy.

Whipple's disease is rare chronic disease caused by a bacterial infection. The affected bowel is usually swollen with raised, yellowish patches. This can usually be seen during sigmoidoscopy or colonoscopy.

In Crohn's disease, the colon wall may have a "cobblestone" appearance due to the intermittent pattern of affected and nonaffected colonic tissue. This can usually be seen during sigmoidoscopy or colonoscopy.

270. B: The patient may have a rotator cuff tear. X rays may be negative because they can only visualize bones, not muscles, ligaments, or tendons. Magnetic resonance imaging (MRI) can definitively determine whether or not a tear is present.

Not treating the patient is not appropriate, especially if he or she has a significantly limited range of motion. Not all rotator cuff tears require surgery, but further evaluation of the injury is warranted because the patient has a significantly decreased range of motion.

Electromyography (EMG) is used to help diagnose the cause of muscle and nerve disorders. It would not be particularly helpful in this case because the patient has a known history of injury. The patient's nerves and muscles are normal; the problem is with the tendon.

271. C: Compartment syndrome involves muscle swelling due to injury, which causes insufficient or complete lack of blood flow to the affected area. The muscles, blood vessels, and tissues of the body are contained into multiple compartments by the fascia. The fascia do not stretch in response to injury, so if the muscle swells, the pressure inside the compartment increases, which can cut off the blood supply to that area. This can cause pallor of the affected area, decreased or absent pulses, and decreased or absent sensation. A creatine phosphokinase (CPK) test might be high due to the muscle damage that is occurring. Compartment syndrome is a surgical emergency. A fasciotomy is performed to allow the muscle to expand without impinging on the blood flow.

Septic arthritis is the infection of a joint or joints due to an infection in the blood. Patients present with a painful, red joint.

Osgood–Schlatter disease is the swelling of the tibial tubercle, which commonly occurs in pubescent and prepubescent children.

Deep venous thrombus is the presence of a clot in the extremity. Patients may be asymptomatic, or they may develop pain and swelling of the affected extremity.

272. B: The patient has trichomoniasis. It is caused by a protozoal infection of the genitourinary tract. It is a sexually transmitted disease that can cause green, frothy discharge from the penis or vagina, dysuria, pain with sexual intercourse, and strong foul vaginal odor. The treatment of choice is metronidazole.

Metronidazole is an antibiotic used in treating anaerobic bacterial infections; it is also used in the treatment of some parasitic infections.

Azithromycin and Rocephin are antibiotics used for bacterial infections such as gonorrhea (GC)/chlamydia.

Fluconazole is an antifungal medication used to treat yeast infections.

273. A: This patient is displaying signs of *peau d'orange,* a French term meaning "skin of an orange." It is cause by impaired lymphatic drainage and edema caused by advanced inflammatory breast cancer.

An abscess is a localized area of erythema and tenderness with induration and/or fluctuance caused by a collection of pus underneath the skin.

Gynecomastia is the overgrowth of breast tissue in males, most commonly occurring in adolescence.

A fibroadenoma is a firm, rubbery, benign breast mass. It does not cause overlying skin changes.

274. D: Caffeine can cause insomnia, abdominal cramping, and diarrhea, and it may cause food cravings. It should generally be avoided before and during one's menses.

Exercise has been shown in numerous studies to limit feelings of depression and provide extra energy during the day.

Eating nutritious meals and snacks throughout the day can help regulate blood sugar, which can curb binge eating, food cravings, and mood swings due to hyperglycemia or hypoglycemia.

Birth control pills can better regulate hormones, which may alleviate or at least partially reduce mood swings and depression caused by premenstrual syndrome.

275. C: Ceasing to have children will not help prevent cervical cancer.

Cervical cancer is caused by the human papilloma virus (HPV). Limiting one's sexual partners can decrease the risk of exposure to HPV and decrease the risk of developing cervical cancer.

Regular Pap smears and gynecological examinations can help detect any anomalies early.

Tobacco abuse can increase one's risk of developing cervical cancer by up to five times more than someone who does not smoke.

276. B: Beriberi is caused by a thiamine deficiency primarily seen in developing or underdeveloped countries. Symptoms may include muscle weakness or paralysis due to damaged nerves, heart failure, pleural effusion, encephalopathy, decreased reflexes, as well as a multitude of other complications. Some of these complications may be permanent if the thiamine deficiency is not corrected quickly.

277. A: Osteoporosis is the presence of decreased bone mineral density in the body, which can lead to persistent pathological fractures, depending on the severity of the disease. There are a multitude of factors that can contribute, such as vitamin D deficiency, tobacco abuse, disease, and being immobile for long periods. A diet rich in calcium and vitamin D can help prevent or at least slow the development of osteoporosis.

278. B: Paget's disease is the abnormal formation and degeneration of bone, usually in a localized area in the body. This may cause bony deformities and pathologic fractures. There is no cure, but there are medications that can slow the progression of the disease and help minimize complications.

Wilms' tumor is the most common renal tumor in pediatric patients.

Osteosarcoma is a type of bone cancer commonly occurring in young children and elderly patients. It can cause pathologic fractures, but it does not cause bones to be chronically misshapen.

Septic arthritis is the infection of a joint or joints due to an infection in the blood. Patients present with a painful, red joint.

279. C: Placental abruption (abruptio placentae) is the complete separation of the placenta, causing bright-red vaginal bleeding, abdominal and/or back pain, and severe contractions.

Placenta previa commonly presents with painless, bright-red vaginal bleeding at the end of the second trimester or the beginning of the third trimester. It is due to a low-lying placenta. As the uterus enlarges, it may push up against the placenta, causing a small part to tear and bright-red bleeding occurs.

Endometriosis is the presence of uterine cells/uterine lining in other areas of the body causing dysmenorrhea, pain with intercourse, and infertility.

Premature rupture of the membranes is when a woman's water breaks prior to the onset of labor.

280. D: This patient most likely has an anterior cruciate ligament tear. In the Lachman test, the patient has his knee flexed at 30°, and the examiner pulls on the tibia anteriorly to see if there is any displacement. If there is anterior displacement, the Lachman test is positive. A magnetic resonance imaging (MRI) scan of the knee is warranted to confirm the diagnosis.

281. C: A Galeazzi fracture is a fracture of the mid or distal radius and dislocation of the radioulnar joint.
A Monteggia fracture is a fracture of the ulna and dislocation of the radius.
A Le Fort fracture is a fracture of the maxilla; this type of fracture has four categories based on severity.
A Colles' fracture is fracture and dorsal displacement of the distal radius. It is commonly referred to as a "dinner-fork deformity" on x-ray.

282. D: A boxer's fracture is the fracture and possible displacement of the fourth or fifth metacarpal, usually following a trauma with a closed fist.
A Colles' fracture is a fracture and dorsal displacement of the distal radius. It is commonly referred to as a "dinner-fork deformity" on x-ray.
A Lisfranc fracture is the fracture and dislocation of one or more of the metatarsals.
A Hangman's fracture is a fracture through the C2, usually following a high-impact trauma or a hanging.

283. C: A completed abortion is when the miscarriage has occurred and the product of conception (POC) has left the body.
Dysmenorrhea is painful or uncomfortable menses.
Abdominal pain and vaginal bleeding may occur in a threatened abortion, but the fetus is still viable. It may be a sign that a miscarriage may occur. However, a woman who experiences a threatened abortion may still deliver a healthy, full-term child.
An incomplete abortion is when the body has expelled only some of the POC. If the patient does not spontaneously expel the POC in the next one to two weeks, medications or dilation and curettage may be performed to remove the rest to prevent infection.

284. B: An ileus is when the bowel has impaired peristalsis. This condition usually occurs after abdominal surgery or disease. The bowel appears to be distended on x ray or computed tomography (CT) scan, but there is no evidence of obstruction.
Toxic megacolon is the pathologic distension of the colon. It is a complication during or following *Clostridium difficile* colitis, although is also may be seen with other diseases such as Crohn's disease.
Irritable bowel syndrome (IBS) is the presence of bowel disturbances without the presence of disease or pathology. Imaging studies are normal. It is commonly linked to anxiety and stress.
Gastroesophageal reflux disease (GERD) is caused by the improper closing of the lower esophageal sphincter, causing chest pain, abdominal pain, burning sensation in the throat, and halitosis.

285. A: Giardiasis, also known as "traveler's diarrhea," is caused by protozoa found in infected water supplies. Signs and symptoms may include profuse watery diarrhea, which may be bloody; nausea; vomiting; abdominal cramping; and fever. The main concern is dehydration, so the patient must be advised to keep hydrated. Other remedies may include ondansetron to prevent nausea, metronidazole to help combat the infection, and loperamide to alleviate the diarrhea.
Furosemide is not an appropriate treatment because as a diuretic its job is to remove fluid from the body, which would only accelerate the development of dehydration.

286. C: Serum calcium is an ineffective test in the workup of lactose intolerance. The test can be normal, and a patient may have lactose intolerance. Lactose intolerance is the body's inability to digest lactose. The undigested lactose can cause flatulence, abdominal cramping, and diarrhea. It is a largely clinical diagnosis, but the other choices given may be ordered to confirm the suspected diagnosis. It is rarely a serious condition.

287. D: A serum beta human chorionic gonadotropin (hCG) test should be ordered to monitor the progression of choriocarcinoma and its response to therapy. It is an abnormal overgrowth of the cells that

normally cover the placenta. It may occur after an ectopic pregnancy, a normal pregnancy, or a planned or spontaneous abortion. Because the placenta produces beta HCG, serial beta HCG levels help monitor the progression or regression of the disease.

A complete blood count is nonspecific and ineffective at monitoring choriocarcinoma.

Bence Jones proteins are found in the urine and may be diagnostic of multiple myeloma.

A computed tomography (CT) scan may help show the size of the tumor and if metastases are present, but ordering several of them would be unwise because it exposes the patient to a significant amount of radiation.

288. C: Antibiotics do not play a role in treating leiomyomas, or uterine fibroids. Fibroids are benign growths that may cause dysmenorrhea, menorrhagia, pain with sexual intercourse, abdominal cramping, and urinary frequency.

Iron supplements help prevent anemia that may be caused by menorrhagia.

Nonsteroidal anti-inflammatory drugs (NSAIDs) can alleviate symptoms of dysmenorrhea and pain with sexual intercourse.

Birth control pills can help regulate hormones and alleviate dysmenorrhea and menorrhagia.

289. D: This patient has endometriosis. Endometriosis is the presence of uterine cells/uterine lining in other areas of the body, causing dysmenorrhea, dysuria, leg cramping, pain with intercourse, and infertility. Imaging studies such as an ultrasound may be normal. Laparoscopy can make the definitive diagnosis.

Dystocia is difficult childbirth.

Fibroids/leiomyomas are benign growths or tumors that may cause dysmenorrhea, menorrhagia, pain with sexual intercourse, abdominal cramping, and urinary frequency. Fibroids large enough to cause symptoms are generally seen on pelvic ultrasound.

Choriocarcinoma is an abnormal overgrowth of the cells that normally cover the placenta. Patients may experience abdominal pain and bleeding. It may occur after an ectopic pregnancy, a normal pregnancy, or a planned or spontaneous abortion. Because the placenta produces beta human chorionic gonadotropin (hCG), a serum HCG or urine pregnancy test will be positive. A mass is usually seen on ultrasound.

290. C: There is no surgery to improve sciatica because the sciatic nerve cannot be removed or resected. The sciatic nerve runs down the lower back and down each of the legs, providing sensation to the lower extremities. The nerve can become inflamed or impinged due to degeneration of the spine, disease, or trauma.

The mainstays of treatment for sciatica are pain medications (such as nonsteroidal anti-inflammatory drugs [NSAIDs], narcotics, and muscle relaxers), ice or heat, and physical therapy.

291. A: Systemic lupus erythematous is an autoimmune disorder that causes inflammation in the joints and organs. There are multiple signs and symptoms, such as polyarthralgia, hair loss, and oral ulcerations, but one of the most unique signs is a malar rash. The malar rash is a butterfly-shaped rash that covers the nose and cheeks.

Paget's disease is the abnormal formation and degeneration of bone, usually in a localized area in the body. This condition may cause bony deformities and pathologic fractures.

Polymyositis is the appearance of bilateral muscle weakness and wasting due to immune disorders or disease.

Huntington's disease is a progressive neurological disorder caused by an autosomal-dominant chromosomal abnormality, which usually occurs in the third or fourth decade of life. Signs include progressive decline in cognitive function; ataxic gait; and uncoordinated, jerky body movements.

292. A: Antibiotics do not play a role in treatment of a small-bowel obstruction. If it is a partial obstruction, conservative management is attempted first. Patients are kept nothing-by-mouth (NPO) status and placed on intravenous (IV) fluid hydration. A nasogastric tube is placed to help decompress the bowel, and antiemetic medications such as Zofran are given as needed for nausea and vomiting.

293. A: Irritable bowel syndrome (IBS) is the presence of bowel disturbances without the presence of disease or pathology. It is commonly linked to anxiety and stress.
In Crohn's disease, the colon wall may have a "cobblestone" appearance due to the intermittent pattern of affected and nonaffected colonic tissue. Ulcerative colitis usually affects continuous stretches of the colon and rectum. The abnormalities of the mucosa can be seen via colonoscopy and imaging studies.
Toxic megacolon is the pathologic distension of the colon seen on CT scan or an x ray of the pelvis. It is a complication during or following *Clostridium difficile* colitis, although it also may be seen with other diseases, such as Crohn's disease.

294. B: Antibiotics are used to treat pelvic inflammatory disease (PID) because it is caused by a bacterial infection. The number-one cause of PID is venereal disease, most notably, gonorrhea and chlamydia. Untreated sexually transmitted diseases may lead to pelvic inflammatory disease, which is the primary preventable cause of infertility. Approximately 10% to 15% of PID cases are caused by illnesses such as appendicitis or pelvic procedures such as dilation and curettage, abortion, or childbirth.

295. D: Corticosteroids are the treatment of choice for polymyositis. Polymyositis is the appearance of bilateral muscle weakness and wasting due to immune disorders or disease. A high creatinine phosphokinase (CPK), a positive muscle biopsy, an elevated white blood cell count, a positive electromyography (EMG), and a history of bilateral muscle weakness with no known cause help confirm the suspected diagnosis. Administration of high-dose steroids may completely reverse the signs and symptoms in most patients.

296. A: Spondylolisthesis is a condition in which the vertebra slips out of place, causing pain or discomfort. The primary cause for this condition is degenerative disease, but it may also be caused by strenuous activity, trauma, or congenital defect. Most treatments include conservative measures such as pain medication, physical therapy, and supportive braces. For severe symptoms or significant disc displacement, surgery may be warranted.

297. C: The withdrawal method involves the male partner pulling out prior to ejaculation. This method has a higher failure rate than the use of intrauterine devices, birth control pills, and condoms, even when it is performed consistently. It is believed that some semen enters the vagina prior to ejaculation, which can result in unwanted pregnancy.

298. D: Methotrexate is an antimetabolite used to treat cancer, autoimmune disorders such as lupus or rheumatoid arthritis, and medical abortions.
Metronidazole is an antibiotic used in treating anaerobic bacterial infections; it is also an amebicide and antiprotozoal medication.
Meropenem is a strong broad-spectrum antibiotic used to treat anaerobic, gram-positive, and gram-negative bacteria.
Metformin is an antihyperglycemic medication used in the treatment of diabetes.

299. B: Though the exact cause of osteoarthritis is unknown, it is related to aging and degenerative disease. Cartilage is a rubbery substance that helps cushion and protect bones. As cartilage gets worn away with age and overuse, the bones begin to rub against each other, causing pain and inflammation. Strenuous activity, multiple fractures, and obesity also play roles in the development of osteoarthritis.

300. A: Kyphosis is an abnormal curvature of the spine, usually due to degenerative disease, but may also be due to trauma, bony diseases such as spina bifida or Paget's disease, and tumors. If the curvature is severe enough, surgery may be warranted, but usually the treatment is conservative management.

Cauda equina syndrome can be caused by disease, trauma, or infection. It affects the nerve roots from L1 to L5 and S1 to S5, which can cause motor dysfunction, urinary retention, saddle anesthesias, among other neurological issues.

Avascular necrosis occurs when there is insufficient or complete lack of blood flow to the bone, causing death of the bone cells. Patients may complain of a painful joint that may or may not be swollen.

The sciatic nerve runs down the lower back and down each of the legs, providing sensation to the lower extremities. The nerve can become inflamed or impinged due to degeneration of the spine, disease, or trauma. It does not cause an abnormal curvature of the spine.

# Practice Test #2

## Practice Questions

1. A 46-year-old man arrives at your family practice office as a new patient since he just moved to the area. His only complaint is soreness in his legs for the past few weeks. He says that his previous primary care provider had recently started him on several new medications. Which of the following medications is likely causing his reported symptom?
   a. Lisinopril
   b. Atorvastatin
   c. Naproxen
   d. Niacin

2. A 64-year-old African-American man with no prior history of cancer asks if he should have a blood test to check for prostate cancer. Since your practice uses the most recent United States Preventive Services Task Force (USPSTF) guidelines, what do you do?
   a. Order a prostate-specific antigen (PSA) test since he is older than 55 years
   b. Do not order a PSA test since he is African American and at lower risk for prostate cancer
   c. Order a PSA test since his brother had prostate cancer
   d. Do not order a PSA test since the harm outweighs the benefit of screening

3. A 25-year-old woman arrives in your urgent care facility with a bright red left sclera. She denies any eye trauma. The review of symptoms is negative besides the patient reporting constipation. How do you treat this patient?
   a. Prescribe antibiotics for 1 week.
   b. Refer her to an ophthalmologist for further evaluation.
   c. Advise her that the condition will likely resolve on its own.
   d. Give a steroid shot today to reduce inflammation.

4. A 43-year-old woman with a history of cocaine dependence presents to your office complaining of stress. She says that for the past 3 months, she has been worrying excessively about her job, finances, relationships, and other daily matters. She denies depressed mood. She would like to start a medication to help with her symptoms. What is a reasonable choice of medication to start?
   a. Buspirone
   b. Clonazepam
   c. Bupropion
   d. Doxepin

5. A 56-year-old woman arrives with an itchy rash that has been present for several weeks. On exam, you find small, flat, purplish papules spread primarily over her forearms and back. You decide to do a biopsy, but in the meantime before the results come back, the patient wants to know if she is contagious. What do you tell her based on your suspected diagnosis at this time?
   a. Not contagious anymore since it started several weeks ago
   b. Contagious for the next 2 to 4 days as she starts antibiotics
   c. Not contagious since this is an autoimmune condition
   d. Contagious until the rash is completely cleared

6. What would you expect to hear on exam when listening to the heart of a patient with known severe aortic stenosis?
    a. High-pitched murmur during diastole
    b. Crescendo-decrescendo ejection murmur
    c. Holosystolic murmur at the apex
    d. Rumbling diastolic murmur at the apex

7. A 72-year-old woman with a history of congestive heart failure (CHF) and hypertension arrives in the emergency department with shortness of breath. Her breath sounds are clear, but you notice an irregularly irregular rhythm with auscultation. What does her electrocardiogram (ECG) likely show?
    a. Myocardial infarction
    b. Pericardial effusion
    c. Atrial fibrillation
    d. Aortic stenosis

8. A 24-year-old woman reports intermittent stomach cramping, diarrhea, and constipation, which has been present for the past 5 years. She has tried cutting out wheat from her diet but did not notice any different in her symptoms. She has had a colonoscopy and endoscopy that had normal results. What is the most likely diagnosis?
    a. Celiac disease
    b. Crohn disease
    c. Irritable bowel syndrome
    d. Ulcerative colitis

9. A 35-year-old woman has fatigue and generalized weakness. She is mildly tachycardic with cool skin, but otherwise the exam is normal. You suspect she is anemic and would like to figure out the cause. Which of the following is NOT a test you would typically order for an initial work-up?
    a. Complete blood cell count (CBC)
    b. Fecal occult blood testing
    c. Complete metabolic panel (CMP)
    d. Bone marrow biopsy

10. A 46-year-old man arrives in the emergency department with confusion. He had previously been diagnosed with AIDS but has not recently been taking antiretrovirals or prophylactic antibiotics. A ring-enhancing lesion is seen on head computed tomography (CT). What is causing his current presentation?
    a. Toxoplasmosis
    b. Kaposi sarcoma
    c. *Pneumocystis jiroveci*
    d. *Mycobacterium avium* complex

11. A 9-year-old boy has an itchy right ear. On exam, you see discharge and pain is elicited with palpation of the tragus. There is no evidence of cellulitis. The patient reports that he has been doing a lot of swimming. How would you treat this patient?
    a. Give a steroid injection.
    b. Prescribe topical antibiotics and steroids.
    c. Prescribe oral antibiotics.
    d. Give an antibiotic injection.

12. You are examining a 6 month old and are only able to palpate one testis in the scrotum. You discuss surgical intervention with the mother. What are the risks if the condition is left untreated?
   a. Possible concurrent inguinal hernia
   b. Decreased fertility
   c. Increased risk of testicular cancer
   d. All of the above

13. An 11-year-old boy arrives in urgent care after falling out of a tree and reaching out to break his fall. On exam, you note tenderness in the "anatomical snuff box" area. You decide to do an x-ray. Which of the following bones do you suspect may be fractured?
   a. Hamate
   b. Triquetrum
   c. Scaphoid
   d. Pisiform

14. A 10-year-old boy arrives in your office for a routine checkup. He is found to have a body mass index (BMI) higher than the 95th percentile. There is a history of cardiovascular disease and hypertension in the family. Which of the following tests should you order first?
   a. CBC and C-reactive protein (CRP)
   b. ECG
   c. Liver function tests (LFTs) and lipid panel
   d. Polysomnography

15. What part of the brain is abnormal in a 72-year-old patient who has a stooped posture, shuffling gait, pill-rolling tremor, and small handwriting?
   a. Pineal body
   b. Medulla oblongata
   c. Cerebellar peduncle
   d. Substantia nigra

16. A 26-year-old man reports a slightly painful and itchy red bump on the outside of his lip. His review of systems is otherwise negative. On exam, you see a small cluster of vesicles on the vermillion border. How do you counsel this patient?
   a. Advise him to be cautious because this condition can spread with or without active lesions
   b. Provide education about how this is linked to his previous chickenpox infection
   c. Tell him that this condition can only be spread by contact with blood
   d. Relieve his concerns by letting him know that the infection does not recur

17. A 57-year-old man was recently admitted to the hospital with shortness of breath, cough, and night sweats. His sputum smear shows acid-fast bacilli. All of the following are risk factors for the development of this disease EXCEPT:
   a. Being a health care worker
   b. Working in a chemical factory
   c. Living in the same household as someone with this disease
   d. Living in poverty

18. Which of the following medications stimulates pancreatic beta cell insulin secretion, thus lowering plasma glucose level?
    a. Acarbose
    b. Metformin
    c. Pioglitazone
    d. Glyburide

19. A temporal artery biopsy can confirm the diagnosis of which condition listed below?
    a. Polyarteritis nodosa
    b. Takayasu arteritis
    c. Giant cell arteritis
    d. Polymyalgia rheumatica

20. A newborn has been in the intensive care unit (ICU) because of cyanotic spells and poor growth. A systolic murmur is heard with auscultation and a boot-shaped heart is seen on x-ray. What is the most likely diagnosis?
    a. Tetralogy of Fallot
    b. Persistent truncus arteriosus
    c. Transposition of the great arteries
    d. Hypoplastic left heart syndrome

21. A previously healthy 2 year old is brought to the emergency department with recurrent and worsening abdominal pain. During your exam, the child passes stool that looks like currant jelly. You note abdominal tenderness and guarding. What are you most concerned about?
    a. Pyloric stenosis
    b. Meconium ileus
    c. Necrotizing enterocolitis
    d. Intussusception

22. A 17-year-old soccer player arrives after a game with knee pain. He says that another player ran into him. On exam, you note swelling and joint line tenderness. McMurray test is positive. Lachman test is negative. Based on this history and exam, what is your diagnosis?
    a. Osteoarthritis
    b. Anterior cruciate ligament tear
    c. Lateral collateral ligament tear
    d. Meniscus tear

23. What would you expect to find in the cerebrospinal fluid (CSF) from a lumbar puncture of a patient with acute bacterial meningitis?
    a. Elevated pressure, neutrophils 2000/mcL, glucose 80 mg/dL, protein 40 mg/dL
    b. Normal pressure, neutrophils 2000/mcL, glucose 40 mg/dL, protein 100 mg/dL
    c. Elevated pressure, neutrophils 2000/mcL, glucose 40 mg/dL, protein 100 mg/dL
    d. Decreased pressure, neutrophils 2000/mcL, glucose 80 mg/dL, protein 40 mg/dL

24. You are examining an ECG that shows dropped P waves. What is the most likely diagnosis?
    a. Sick sinus syndrome
    b. Wandering atrial pacemaker
    c. Wolff-Parkinson-White syndrome
    d. None of the above

25. During an annual physical, a 50-year-old man has in-office blood pressure readings of 145/92 and 143/89, taken 5 minutes apart. He has previously tried diet and exercise with no change in blood pressure. He does not have a history of kidney problems or heart attack. According to the Joint National Committee, which medication should he be started on?
a. Metoprolol
b. Nifedipine
c. Hydrochlorothiazide
d. Lisinopril

26. A 34-year-old man arrives in the emergency department after being hit in the face. He complains of double vision. You notice bruising around his right eye. On x-ray, you see a "teardrop sign." Which muscle is likely affected?
a. Inferior rectus
b. Superior oblique
c. Lateral rectus
d. Superior rectus

27. A generally healthy 20-year-old man has had 1 week of pruritus that seems to be worse at night. His girlfriend has been having the same problem. On exam, you notice erythematous papules and scaly lines between his fingers and also around his waistline. How do you treat this?
a. No medications now, reevaluate in 3 days
b. Oral doxycycline for 1 week
c. Permethrin cream applied to the whole body
b. Miconazole on the affected areas

28. All of the following x-ray findings would raise suspicion for abuse EXCEPT:
a. 9 year old with distal radius fracture
b. 13 year old with rib fracture
c. 5 year old with spiral fracture of the femur
d. 2 year old with skull fracture across a suture line

29. A 16 year old wakes up in the middle of the night with left testicular pain. He comes to the emergency department where he is found to have a fever and an absent cremasteric reflex on the affected side. What is the most likely diagnosis?
a. Varicocele
b. Testicular cancer
c. Testicular torsion
d. Hydrocele

30. What would you expect with a positive obturator sign when performing an exam on a patient with suspected appendicitis?
a. Increased pain when passively extending the right hip
b. Increased pain when passively flexing and externally rotating the right hip
c. Increased pain when passively extending the left hip
d. Increased pain when passively flexing and internally rotating the right hip

31. A 30-year-old man arrives in the emergency department with left ankle pain, which started during a basketball game when he landed after going up for a shot. You determine that he has a sprain and would like to prescribe tramadol for short-term management of his pain. However, you need to counsel him on drug interactions because he is also taking which of the following other medications?
    a. Omeprazole
    b. Ibuprofen
    c. Sertraline
    d. Valacyclovir

32. A 3-year-old girl has sneezing, watery eyes, and a worsening cough. She has been having bouts of coughing followed by high-pitched deep inspirations. She has started to vomit as well. Swab shows gram negative coccobacilli. What is the causative organism?
    a. *Moraxella catarrhalis*
    b. *Bordetella pertussis*
    c. *Streptococcus pneumoniae*
    d. *Staphylococcus aureus*

33. Which of the following conditions would require the most immediate treatment?
    a. Chalazion
    b. Entropion
    c. Peritonsillar abscess
    d. Aphthous ulcer

34. According to the United States Preventive Services Task Force, screening for abdominal aortic aneurysm could be appropriate for all of the following patients EXCEPT:
    a. 65-year-old man with history of smoking
    b. 72-year-old man with no history of smoking
    c. 74-year-old man with history of smoking
    d. 68-year-old woman with history of smoking

35. A 34-year-old woman has fatigue, fever, headache, and joint pain. She reports that she just returned from camping in Maryland. On exam, you notice a large macule on her back with central clearing. What is the most likely diagnosis?
    a. Rocky Mountain spotted fever
    b. Erythema infectiosum
    c. Lyme disease
    d. Syphilis

36. What are the characteristics of an indirect inguinal hernia?
    a. Congenital protrusion through the inguinal ring into inguinal canal
    b. Protrusion through weak spot of inguinal canal
    c. Occurs below inguinal ligament at weak spot of femoral canal
    d. Occurs at umbilical ring through abdominal wall

37. According to the American Congress of Obstetricians and Gynecologists (ACOG), which of the following average risk patients should have a Pap smear now?
    a. 18 year old who has been sexually active for the past year
    b. 28 year old who had a normal Pap smear 1 year ago
    c. 60 year old who had a normal Pap smear 5 years ago
    d. 66 year old whose last 3 Pap smears in 10 years have been normal

- 111 -

38. You are seeing a patient whose thyroid-stimulating hormone (TSH) is 6.3 and free $T_4$ is 0.4. What is your next step?
    a. Use beta-blockers to control symptoms
    b. Start iodine therapy
    c. Refer to surgery
    d. Start levothyroxine

39. A 63-year-old male Vietnam combat veteran has a 5-year history of flashbacks, extreme irritability, and increased startle response. Your working diagnosis is posttraumatic stress disorder. You expect him to report that he is doing all of the following EXCEPT:
    a. Waking up at night to check door locks and survey the house
    b. Attending more military events and talking about his experiences
    c. Having frequent nightmares about combat situations
    d. Feeling detached from family and friends

40. In the treatment of hypertension, which of the following diuretics acts by inhibiting chloride reabsorption in the ascending loop of Henle?
    a. Furosemide
    b. Triamterene
    c. Spironolactone
    d. Acetazolamide

41. An overweight 12-year-old boy has pain and swelling below his right kneecap. He does not remember a specific injury but is actively involved in sports. What is the most likely diagnosis?
    a. Slipped capital femoral epiphysis
    b. Sever disease
    c. Osgood-Schlatter disease
    d. Scheuermann disease

42. A 35-year-old man has an itchy, red rash in his armpits that has been present for the past 2 days. He often works outside in the heat and is otherwise healthy. What is the best tool to confirm diagnosis given this presentation?
    a. Potassium hydroxide wet mount
    b. Punch biopsy
    c. Tzanck smear
    d. Shave biopsy

43. A 45-year-old woman is concerned that she has developed some varicose veins over the past several months. How do you counsel this patient?
    a. Tell her that nothing can be done since it is strictly genetic.
    b. Advise use of compression stockings since she is on her feet all day.
    c. Tell her that elevating her legs can worsen the discomfort.
    d. Recommend that she see a surgeon since this will be a definitive cure.

44. Which of the following is true about Tourette disorder?
    a. Diagnosis includes motor tics and at least one vocal tic
    b. It is a hereditary condition and more common in males
    c. Comorbid conditions include ADHD and OCD
    d. All of the above

45. A 17 year old arrives in the office with left eye pain and redness. He feels like something is in his eye. He says that he has been sleeping in his contacts for the past week, but took them out earlier this morning. You use fluorescein staining and notice an abrasion but do not see a foreign body. How do you treat this patient?
    a. Immediate copious irrigation
    b. Eye patch for 1 week
    c. Antibiotic ointment for 5 days
    d. Ophthalmic corticosteroids

46. A 28-year-old woman has wrist pain on the thumb side. The Finkelstein test is positive. The tendons of which muscles are affected in this syndrome?
    a. Abductor pollicus longus and extensor pollicus brevis
    b. Extensor carpi radialis brevis and extensor carpi radialis longus
    c. Abductor pollicus longus and extensor pollicus longus
    d. Extensor digitorum and extensor pollicus longus

47. Hepatitis C is most commonly transmitted through which of the following?
    a. Breastfeeding
    b. Sex
    c. Blood
    d. Feces

48. A 25-year-old woman reports that she and her husband have been trying to conceive. They have been having unprotected intercourse for the past 6 months with no resulting pregnancy. How do you help this patient?
    a. Set her up an appointment with an infertility specialist.
    b. Counsel her that infertility is not diagnosed until after 1 year of unprotected intercourse.
    c. Advise that her husband come in for testing.
    d. Order a hysterosalpingography.

49. Which of the following drugs has been linked most strongly with the adverse effect of aplastic anemia?
    a. Phenylephrine
    b. Gentamicin
    c. Cyclobenzaprine
    d. Carbamazepine

50. A 35-year-old woman reports recurrent episodes where she feels dizzy and has ringing in her ears. They usually last several hours accompanied by nausea. She has had several hearing tests over the years that showed varying results. She thinks her mother may have experienced similar symptoms. She denies ear discharge or pain. What is your suspected diagnosis?
    a. Chronic otitis media
    b. Dysfunction of Eustachian tube
    c. Ménière disease
    d. Cholesteatoma

51. A 22-year-old man arrives in the emergency department with sudden onset of shortness of breath. He is otherwise healthy. On exam, you note hyperresonance to percussion and absent breath sounds on the right side. On x-ray, the heart has shifted out of the midline. How do you treat this patient?
    a. Oxygen only
    b. Serial x-rays for monitoring
    c. Catheter drainage
    d. Continuous positive airway pressure (CPAP)

52. A 21-year-old woman has symptoms of dysuria and frequency for the first time. She is not pregnant, and there is no costovertebral angle (CVA) tenderness. The urine dipstick is positive for leukocyte esterase and nitrites. What is the most likely causative organism?
    a. *E. coli*
    b. *Enterobacter*
    c. *Serratia*
    d. *Pseudomonas*

53. Which of the following is NOT a sign of Cushing syndrome?
    a. Thin skin with striae
    b. Central obesity
    c. Decreased hair growth
    d. "Moon face"

54. A 26-year-old man has 3 to 4 cm depigmented irregular patches on his fingertips that have been present for the past 2 months and seem to be growing. What is likely happening to this patient?
    a. Acute infection with a virus
    b. Too much sun exposure
    c. Chronic fungal infection with underlying disease
    d. Loss of skin melanocytes with unclear cause

55. What is considered first-line therapy for hypertrophic cardiomyopathy?
    a. Beta-blockers
    b. Nitrates
    c. Inotropes
    d. Angiotensin-converting enzyme (ACE) inhibitors

56. A toddler has jaw stiffness, headache, and fever 7 days after stepping on a dirty nail. The patient has not received any immunizations. CSF is clear. Which of the following is NOT a usual component of treatment for this condition?
    a. Steroids
    b. Human immune globulin
    c. Metronidazole
    d. Diazepam

57. What is the most frequent complication of performing an endoscopic retrograde cholangiopancreatography (ERCP)?
    a. Aspiration
    b. Pancreatitis
    c. Perforation
    d. Cholangitis

58. How does donepezil work in the treatment of Alzheimer disease?
   a. Acetyl/butyrylcholinesterase inhibitor
   b. Acetylcholinesterase inhibitor
   c. Cholinesterase and nicotinic receptor stimulation modulator
   d. Glutamate antagonist

59. A 32-year-old woman has a 1-week history of runny nose, cough, and fever. On exam, you note tenderness to palpation of the forehead. What is the most likely diagnosis?
   a. Sinusitis
   b. Allergic rhinitis
   c. Parotitis
   d. Nasal polyps

60. A 46-year-old man arrives in the emergency department with depressed mood, insomnia, low energy, and poor concentration for the past month. He has been having intermittent thoughts about suicide, but has not thought of a specific plan. He says that he does not want to commit suicide because of his family. He also does not want to have to stay in the hospital. What is the most appropriate course of action?
   a. Admit him to the hospital involuntarily since you think he is an imminent danger to himself.
   b. Advise that he find a psychologist since mental health issues are not treated in the emergency department.
   c. Send him home with a month's supply of a mood stabilizer to try out for his symptoms.
   d. Discharge him with a low-dose antidepressant and make a close psychiatry follow-up appointment.

61. For patients who have frequent clots or cannot take anticoagulants, where are Greenfield filters implanted in order to prevent pulmonary emboli?
   a. Superior vena cava
   b. Femoral vein
   c. Inferior vena cava
   d. Pulmonary artery

62. A 29-year-old man has had right elbow pain for the past 3 weeks. On exam, you note pain with wrist extension and tenderness over the lateral humeral epicondyle. There is no edema. What is the most likely diagnosis based on this information?
   a. "Golfer's elbow"
   b. Olecranon bursitis
   c. Ulnar collateral ligament tear
   d. "Tennis elbow"

63. You are seeing a 55-year-old man for routine follow-up. He has diabetes mellitus (DM) and peripheral vascular disease (PVD), and is a smoker. What is his low-density lipoprotein (LDL) goal?
   a. < 100 mg/dL
   b. < 130 mg/dL
   c. < 160 mg/dL
   d. < 190 mg/dL

64. A 49-year-old man with a history of diabetes mellitus arrives in the emergency department with shortness of breath and chest pain. He had knee surgery 1 week ago. He is tachycardic and hypotensive, and you note crackles with auscultation of the lungs. Chest x-ray and troponin are normal. What is the most likely diagnosis based on this information?
    a. Pneumonia
    b. Pulmonary embolism (PE)
    c. Acute myocardial infarction (MI)
    d. Congestive heart failure (CHF) exacerbation

65. You diagnose a 10-year-old girl with influenza and prescribe oseltamivir. She has had symptoms for 1 day. How do you counsel the patient's mother with regard to expectations for the medication?
    a. The duration of symptoms will be reduced by 1 day.
    b. Acetaminophen cannot be given concurrently.
    c. The patient will never need to have another influenza vaccine.
    d. The patient should be cured after 1 day.

66. A 25-year-old generally healthy white man has dull testicular pain present for the past 2 weeks. He denies penile discharge, and the scrotum is nonerythematous. He is negative for sexually transmitted diseases. What do you suspect?
    a. Spermatocele
    b. Epididymitis
    c. Hydrocele
    d. Testicular cancer

67. Metronidazole can be used to treat which of the following conditions?
    a. Lichen sclerosis
    b. Vulvovaginal candidiasis
    c. Trichomoniasis
    d. Atrophic vaginitis

68. A 32-year-old generally healthy man has had a rash over his back for the past week with itching. On exam, you note multiple rose-colored oval papules spread over the back in a "Christmas tree" distribution. The lesions are somewhat scaly. With further questioning, he remembers initially seeing a single larger lesion on his trunk about a week ago. How do you treat this patient?
    a. Antibiotics for 5 days
    b. Topical antifungal applied over the whole body
    c. No treatment necessary as it will go away on its own
    d. Immunomodulatory drugs long-term

69. Which of the following is true regarding primary hypertension?
    a. Roughly 1 in 3 Americans has it.
    b. Prevalence increases with age.
    c. It occurs more often in black patients.
    d. All of the above

70. You encounter a patient with "saddle anesthesia," which you determine as cauda equina syndrome. Between what vertebral levels is the cauda equina located?
    a. L2 to coccyx
    b. L3 to S5
    c. L5 to coccyx
    d. L1 to S2

71. What is the mechanism of action for ranitidine?
    a. $H_1$ receptor agonist
    b. $H_2$ receptor antagonist
    c. $H_1$ receptor antagonist
    d. $H_2$ receptor agonist

72. In a patient with congestive heart failure (CHF), what might you find on chest x-ray?
    a. Kerley B lines
    b. Decreased heart size
    c. Ground glass appearance
    d. Silhouette sign

73. A 7-year-old boy arrives in the emergency department with rapid onset of sore throat, difficulty swallowing, and fever. On exam, you note that he is drooling, leaning over, and having a hard time breathing in. What is the most likely diagnosis?
    a. Pertussis
    b. Pneumonia
    c. Epiglottitis
    d. Respiratory syncytial virus (RSV)

74. Ectopic pregnancies occur most often in which structure?
    a. Uterine interstitium
    b. Fallopian tube
    c. Cervix
    d. Pelvic cavity

75. You encounter a patient who has had several incidences of optic neuritis. What would be the best test to order so that more serious comorbid conditions can be ruled out?
    a. HIV
    b. Lumbar puncture
    c. Reticulocyte count
    d. Magnetic resonance imaging (MRI)

76. A 9-year-old girl with asthma has shortness of breath, chest tightness, and wheezing. She was unable to participate in school sports yesterday. She has been having these symptoms 4 times a week during the day and 3 times a month during the night. She has been using a rescue beta-agonist as needed. What do you recommend next?
    a. Use of rescue beta-agonist more frequently
    b. High-dose inhaled corticosteroid daily
    c. Low-dose inhaled corticosteroid daily
    d. Long-acting beta-agonist

77. You are working with a team to monitor a patient who has been seizing for over 20 minutes. The patient has been given lorazepam, phenytoin, and valproate intravenously but there is no improvement. What is the next step?
    a. Give patient up to 30 minutes total to see if seizure will end
    b. Prepare for surgery
    c. Administration of additional anticonvulsant
    d. Intubation and general anesthesia

78. All of the following are signs of pituitary dwarfism in children EXCEPT:
    a. Height is below the 3rd percentile.
    b. Proportions are not normal.
    c. Skeletal maturation is more than 2 years behind chronologic age.
    d. The child fails to begin pubertal development or is delayed.

79. You are treating a patient with quetiapine for mood stabilization and psychotic symptoms. Which of the following need to be ordered regularly?
    a. HbA$_{1c}$
    b. Platelet count
    c. TSH
    d. Kidney function tests

80. What would you expect to see on the ECG of a patient having an acute MI?
    a. Normal T waves
    b. ST segment abnormality
    c. PR interval elongation
    d. Ventricular premature beats

81. A 67-year-old woman has had bilateral knee pain for the past 3 months. She does not recall any specific injury. On exam, you note mild swelling and tenderness. X-rays show joint space narrowing and osteophytes. What do you prescribe this patient?
    a. Steroids
    b. Nonsteroidal anti-inflammatory drugs (NSAIDs)
    c. Narcotics
    d. Muscle relaxants

82. What would you expect to find when evaluating a patient with known benign prostatic hyperplasia?
    a. Rubbery prostate with digital rectal exam
    b. Patient report of painful urination
    c. Hard, nodular prostate with digital rectal exam
    d. Fever and elevated white blood cell count (WBC)

83. A 28-year-old man has a complaint of "bumps" on his forehead, which have been present for several months. He does not recall any trauma and says that they are not painful or particularly itchy. On exam, you note a cluster of 2 mm papules that are flesh-colored, smooth, and round, and have a central umbilication. What is the most likely diagnosis?
    a. Milia
    b. Warts
    c. Folliculitis
    d. Molluscum contagiosum

84. What is a risk factor for development of endometriosis?
    a. Lengthened menstrual cycles
    b. Delayed childbearing
    c. Short periods
    d. Multiple pregnancies

85. A 46-year-old man arrives in the emergency department with severe chest pain that is worsened by deep inspiration and relieved by leaning forward. The patient is hypotensive and tachypneic, and you hear a friction rub with auscultation. Echocardiography shows an effusion. How do you treat this patient?
    a. Valvuloplasty
    b. Tube thoracostomy
    c. Pericardiocentesis
    d. Cardiac catheterization

86. At what gestational age are low-risk pregnant women usually screened for diabetes?
    a. 10 to 12 weeks
    b. 28 to 32 weeks
    c. 12 to 16 weeks
    d. 24 to 28 weeks

87. What of the following medications would not be advised for use in a patient with glaucoma?
    a. Amitriptyline
    b. Levothyroxine
    c. Montelukast
    d. Travoprost

88. You are seeing a patient who likely has gout for the first time, but you want to be sure. What do you order to confirm diagnosis?
    a. Uric acid level
    b. Arthrocentesis
    c. X-ray
    d. Erythrocyte sedimentation rate (ESR)

89. Which of the following is NOT true regarding the physiology of cirrhosis?
    a. Progression of fibrosis varies among individuals
    b. New interconnecting vessels form that contribute to portal hypertension
    c. Loss of hepatic function can lead to liver failure
    d. Growth regulators cause hepatocellular hypoplasia

90. Which of the following is true regarding end-of-life issues with cystic fibrosis patients?
    a. Most patients will live into their 50s or 60s.
    b. Lung transplantation is not an option.
    c. Palliative care should be discussed.
    d. All of the above

91. How would you counsel patients regarding prevention of oral cancer?
    a. Advise them to avoid spicy foods.
    b. Educate them about how this condition is primarily genetic.
    c. Tell them to avoid smoking as this is the biggest risk factor.
    d. Recommend yearly biopsies for screening.

92. A 36-year-old woman arrives in the emergency department with complaints of progressive bilateral lower extremity weakness and tingling over the past week. She says that she had an upper respiratory tract infection 3 weeks ago. On exam, you cannot elicit patellar reflexes. What is the most likely diagnosis?
    a. Stroke
    b. Myasthenia gravis
    c. Amyotrophic lateral sclerosis
    d. Guillain-Barré syndrome

93. A 27-year-old generally healthy woman has mildly painful/itchy clusters of pustules around her nose and mouth. Honey-colored crusts are present over an erythematous base. How do you treat this patient?
    a. Hydrocortisone cream
    b. Mupirocin ointment
    c. Oral nystatin
    d. Retinol cream

94. What is a potential finding in a CT scan of a patient with schizophrenia?
    a. Decreased volume of third ventricle
    b. Larger amygdala
    c. Reduction in brain volume
    d. Increased gray matter

95. Where does a Wilms tumor occur?
    a. Kidney
    b. Liver
    c. Pancreas
    d. Colon

96. What is a common manifestation of multiple myeloma?
    a. Liver insufficiency
    b. Skin rash
    c. Shortness of breath
    d. Bone pain

97. A 22-year-old man has dysuria and penile discharge. He had unprotected sex about a week ago. What do you prescribe this patient?
    a. Azithromycin
    b. Nitrofurantoin
    c. Vancomycin
    d. Bacitracin

98. When may a surgical consult be appropriate for management of hemorrhoids?
    a. After hemorrhoid has been present for 6 months
    b. With patients who have external hemorrhoids
    c. When hemorrhoids fail to respond to more conservative measures
    d. After patient begins experiencing pain

99. A 56-year-old woman arrives in the emergency department with left lower quadrant pain and fever. On exam, you note abdominal tenderness and guarding. WBC is elevated. Based on this information, what do you suspect is wrong with this patient?
   a. Cholecystitis
   b. Diverticulitis
   c. Appendicitis
   d. Colon cancer

100. Which of the following is a long-acting insulin used in the treatment of diabetes?
   a. Aspart
   b. Glargine
   c. Lispro
   d. NPH

101. A 36-year-old man has had fever and fatigue for the past week. He had a dental procedure 2 weeks ago. On exam, you note splinter hemorrhages under the nails and a heart murmur. What do you suspect?
   a. Acute bacterial endocarditis
   b. Pericarditis
   c. Aortic aneurysm
   d. Hypertrophic cardiomyopathy

102. An 18 year old arrives in your office because she has never had a menstrual period. She has never been pregnant. What could be happening with this patient?
   a. Excessive luteinizing hormone (LH) secretion
   b. Decreased gonadotropin secretion
   c. Excessive estrogen level
   d. Decreased testosterone level

103. A 45-year-old woman arrives in your office with complaints of a progressive growth on her right eye. She reports foreign body sensation. On exam, you see a triangular shaped growth from the nasal side of her right eye extending to the edge of her cornea. Her vision is intact. What test do you need to order for confirmation of diagnosis?
   a. MRI
   b. ESR
   c. Herpes simplex virus (HSV)
   d. None of the above

104. You have a patient who takes isosorbide dinitrate for angina pectoris. Which of the following medications would be contraindicated for this patient?
   a. Aspirin
   b. Metoprolol
   c. Sildenafil
   d. Esomeprazole

105. According to the Centers for Disease Control and Prevention, at what age should a healthy nonsmoking adult receive the pneumococcal vaccine if they received their first dose as a child?
   a. 65
   b. 60
   c. 55
   d. 50

- 121 -

106. You are examining a 67-year-old patient who has had a progressive hand tremor. You note a bilateral, slow tremor that is absent at rest. How can you treat this patient?
    a. Phenytoin
    b. Primidone
    c. Terazosin
    d. Levodopa

107. A 31-year-old woman has a 2 cm soft, round swelling on the dorsal side of her left wrist. She does not remember any specific trauma but reports that it has increased in size over the past few months. What is the most likely diagnosis?
    a. Gout
    b. Tenosynovitis
    c. Colles fracture
    d. Ganglion cyst

108. What is a risk factor for the development of actinic keratosis?
    a. Smoking
    b. Frequent sun exposure
    c. Long-term use of retinoid medications
    d. Poor hygiene

109. Which of the following patients is most likely to develop mastitis?
    a. 18-year-old woman who has fibrocystic disease
    b. 58-year-old woman with remote history of breast cancer
    c. 44-year-old man with gynecomastia
    d. 26-year-old woman who is breastfeeding

110. A discrete 1 cm lung nodule is incidentally found on the chest x-ray of a 46-year-old nonsmoking man. There are no other x-rays for comparison. The patient is asymptomatic. What is the best next step?
    a. Oncology referral
    b. Chest CT
    c. Lung biopsy
    d. X-ray in 1 year

111. A 70-year-old woman was found to have osteoporosis on dual-energy x-ray absorptiometry (DEXA) screening. You do not want this patient's condition to worsen, so you recommend all of the following EXCEPT:
    a. Taking a calcium and vitamin D supplement
    b. Decreasing physical activity
    c. Minimizing caffeine and alcohol intake
    d. Starting a bisphosphonate medication

112. A 41-year-old man was admitted to the psychiatry unit for treatment of alcohol dependence. What medication do you use to treat acute withdrawal symptoms?
    a. Lorazepam
    b. Clozapine
    c. Divalproex
    d. Methadone

113. What medication can be given to a premature infant with a patent ductus arteriosus?
   a. Pregabalin
   b. Peginterferon
   c. Epinephrine
   d. Indomethacin

114. You order a hearing test for an elderly patient who you suspect suffers from presbyacusis. Which frequencies would you expect to be affected?
   a. Low
   b. Medium
   c. High
   d. None

115. Which of the following is true regarding both dilated and restrictive cardiomyopathies?
   a. Systolic dysfunction is predominant.
   b. There are numerous potential etiologies.
   c. Only the left ventricle is affected.
   d. Patients have chest pain.

116. A 35-year-old man arrives in the emergency department with intermittent severe back pain, dysuria, and nausea. He is afebrile. Microscopic hematuria is seen on urinalysis. What is the most likely diagnosis based on this information?
   a. Benign prostatic hypertrophy
   b. Pyelonephritis
   c. Prostatitis
   d. Nephrolithiasis

117. A 25-year-old generally healthy woman has a cough, runny nose, and sore throat. She denies headache or itchy eyes. She is afebrile and lung sounds are normal. Mild erythema is seen in the posterior pharynx. What is the most likely diagnosis?
   a. Allergic rhinitis
   b. Sinusitis
   c. Acute bronchitis
   d. Pneumonia

118. Which of the following conditions will have a positive Murphy sign?
   a. Cholecystitis
   b. Pancreatitis
   c. Appendicitis
   d. Peptic ulcer disease

119. How do you manage a patient with abruptio placentae at 35 weeks who presents with vaginal bleeding and with fetal distress?
   a. Prompt delivery
   b. Magnesium
   c. Bed rest
   d. Oxygen

120. Which of the following drug classes is most likely responsible for a patient developing Stevens-Johnson syndrome?
   a. Antipsychotics
   b. Antibiotics
   c. Antihypertensives
   d. Antivirals

121. A 78 year old with dementia is brought in the office by his daughter for routine follow-up. He is disheveled and smells of urine. You notice several bruises on his back. What is the most important step in management of this patient?
   a. Referring to a social worker
   b. Ordering home health services
   c. Educating daughter on care of patient
   d. Contacting Adult Protective Services

122. A 10-year-old girl arrives for an annual physical accompanied by her mother. She is generally healthy although describes anal itching that is worse at night. How do you treat this patient based on your suspected diagnosis?
   a. Fluconazole
   b. Hydrocortisone
   c. Mebendazole
   d. Amoxicillin

123. What is the physiology of hyaline membrane disease in neonates?
   a. Chronic lung injury due to mechanical ventilation
   b. Aspiration of meconium
   c. Bacterial infection of the trachea
   d. Deficiency of pulmonary surfactant

124. Which of the following is true regarding ST elevation MI (STEMI) and non-ST elevation MI (NSTEMI)?
   a. Emergency percutaneous coronary intervention is always necessary.
   b. Patients present with the same symptoms.
   c. Both involve transmural ischemia.
   d. All of the above

125. How do you counsel a patient with gout about how to prevent flare-ups?
   a. Avoid alcohol.
   b. Eat more red meat.
   c. Avoid NSAIDs.
   d. Decrease physical activity.

126. A 54-year-old man with hypertension arrives in the emergency department with sudden onset of "ripping" chest pain. Chest x-ray shows a widened mediastinum. What is the most likely diagnosis?
   a. CHF exacerbation
   b. Acute MI
   c. Pericarditis
   d. Aortic dissection

127. You treat a 30-year-old woman for a urinary tract infection with antibiotics. She comes back 2 weeks later and complains of watery diarrhea with mucus and abdominal cramping. She is febrile. What is the most likely causative organism of the diarrhea?
    a. *Salmonella*
    b. *C. difficile*
    c. *Shigella*
    d. *E. coli*

128. All of the following are possible components in the management of strabismus EXCEPT:
    a. Patching of the normal eye
    b. Eyeglasses or contacts
    c. Surgery
    d. Topical mydriatic agents

129. You are examining a 40-year-old woman with fair skin who has generalized facial erythema, telangiectasias, and scattered pustules. She says that she often feels "flushed." What is the most likely diagnosis?
    a. Psoriasis
    b. Rosacea
    c. Erysipelas
    d. Melasma

130. Which of the following patients should NOT receive the influenza vaccination?
    a. 9-month-old male infant
    b. 38-year-old pregnant woman
    c. 24-year-old woman with upper respiratory tract infection and fever
    d. 86-year-old man living in a nursing home

131. What would you expect to find when reviewing lab results of a patient with untreated hypoparathyroidism?
    a. Low calcium
    b. Elevated magnesium
    c. Low TSH
    d. Elevated phosphate

132. You are evaluating a patient with low back pain and want to prescribe him NSAIDs. Which common potential side effect do you need to warn him about?
    a. GI bleed
    b. Decreased thyroid function
    c. Low platelets
    d. Myalgia

133. For women, what is the biggest risk factor for developing breast cancer?
    a. Family history of breast cancer
    b. Increasing age
    c. Oral contraceptive use
    d. Early menarche

134. A 4-year-old black boy is treated for a viral upper respiratory tract infection. He returns a week later with jaundice. Lab tests show anemia and reticulocytosis, with Heinz bodies and "bite cells" seen on smear. What is the most likely diagnosis?
   a. Autoimmune hemolytic anemia
   b. Sickle cell anemia
   c. Glucose-6-phosphate dehydrogenase (G6PD) deficiency
   d. Hereditary spherocytosis

135. Name the correct order for blood flow through the heart.
   a. Right atrium, right ventricle, left atrium, left ventricle
   b. Left atrium, left ventricle, right atrium, right ventricle
   c. Right atrium, left atrium, right ventricle, left ventricle
   d. Left atrium, right atrium, right ventricle, left ventricle

136. A 40-year-old generally healthy man arrives for routine follow-up and reports that it is getting harder for him to exercise without feeling short of breath. On exam, you note a faint midsystolic murmur near the upper left sternal border. Chest x-ray shows a dilated right atrium. What is the most likely diagnosis?
   a. Coarctation of the aorta
   b. Ventricular septal defect
   c. Patent foramen ovale
   d. Hypoplastic left heart syndrome

137. A 28-year-old man arrives in the emergency department with sudden onset of unilateral, severe headache. There has not been any trauma. You note tearing and rhinorrhea on the affected side. What do you do next?
   a. Order a head CT.
   b. Perform a lumbar puncture.
   c. Order a urine toxicology screen.
   d. Administer 100% oxygen.

138. Which of the following is true regarding erectile dysfunction?
   a. It can be caused by stress or anxiety.
   b. In the United States, 5 to 10 million men are affected.
   c. It is treated with phosphodiesterase inhibitors.
   d. All of the above

139. Which of the following women needs to receive the Rh immune globulin injection?
   a. Rh-positive mother who gave birth to an Rh-positive baby
   b. Rh-negative mother who gave birth to an Rh-negative baby
   c. Rh-positive mother who gave birth to an Rh-negative baby
   d. Rh-negative mother who gave birth to an Rh-positive baby

140. A 60-year-old man has been experiencing intermittent syncopal episodes. He also reports angina and shortness of breath with exertion. On exam, you hear a crescendo-decrescendo ejection murmur. What is the most likely diagnosis?
   a. Mitral stenosis
   b. Aortic stenosis
   c. Mitral regurgitation
   d. Aortic regurgitation

141. You diagnose a patient with Kaposi sarcoma. Out of the following lab tests, which results do you most likely expect to find?
- a. Positive HCV
- b. Reactive RPR
- c. Positive HBsAg
- d. Positive HIV

142. A 17-year-old man has had fatigue for the past 2 weeks. He has also been having fever and sore throat. On exam, you note anterior/posterior cervical lymphadenopathy and splenomegaly. How do you manage this patient based on your suspected diagnosis?
- a. Give antibiotics for 1 week.
- b. Treat supportively.
- c. Administer a steroid injection.
- d. Prescribe antifungals.

143. You are treating a patient who has emphysema with salmeterol. What type of medication is this?
- a. Steroid
- b. Short-acting beta-agonist
- c. Anticholinergic
- d. Long-acting beta-agonist

144. All of the following are true regarding abdominal aortic aneurysms EXCEPT:
- a. Due to weakening of the arterial wall
- b. Typically begin above the renal arteries
- c. Involves the intima, media, and adventitia arterial layers
- d. Generally considered an aneurysm when diameter is 3 cm or more

145. A 25-year-old woman reports lower abdominal pain, vaginal discharge, and irregular bleeding. She has never been pregnant. She has a history of chlamydia. On exam, the cervix is erythematous with visible discharge and motion tenderness. What is the most likely diagnosis?
- a. Endometriosis
- b. Ovarian cyst
- c. Cervical cancer
- d. Pelvic inflammatory disease

146. A 36-year-old man arrives in your office following an accident at work in which he thinks some debris got into his eye. How can you evaluate for corneal abrasions?
- a. Visual field testing
- b. Head CT
- c. Tonometry
- d. Fluorescein staining

147. A 45-year-old man tells you that he has an unreasonable fear of dogs that started about a decade ago after he was attacked by one. Now, he avoids walking on streets where he knows dog owners live. If he sees a dog on TV, he breaks out into sweats and feels anxious. You would like to refer him to a psychologist for therapy. Which therapy modality will be used to treat this patient?
- a. Cognitive processing therapy
- b. Exposure therapy
- c. Psychodynamic therapy
- d. Dialectical behavior therapy

148. Where would you expect a patient with acute pancreatitis to report pain?
   a. Upper abdomen, radiating to the back
   b. Right upper quadrant
   c. Left flank, radiating to lower abdomen
   d. Left lower quadrant

149. A 32-year-old white male reports right knee pain and left hip pain for the past 2 weeks. He has also been having pain with urination and discharge. He had a recent gonorrhea infection. On exam, you note swelling and tenderness in the affected joints. You also notice redness of his eyes. ESR is elevated. What is the most likely diagnosis?
   a. Psoriatic arthritis
   b. Ankylosing spondylitis
   c. Reactive arthritis
   d. Sjögren syndrome

150. You are seeing a patient who has a B-type natriuretic peptide (BNP) level of 680. What condition is this elevated lab usually associated with?
   a. Lung cancer
   b. Congestive heart failure
   c. Pancreatitis
   d. Cirrhosis

151. You see a patient with a history of smoking who has metastatic cancer, with the primary site being a perihilar mass. His condition has been complicated by superior vena cava syndrome. Which type of lung cancer does this patient likely have?
   a. Adenocarcinoma
   b. Small cell lung carcinoma
   c. Large cell lung carcinoma
   d. Squamous cell lung carcinoma

152. A 50-year-old woman has tingling and pain in her hands that is worse at night. She has worked in a job for years where she does a lot of typing. Phalen test is positive. Which nerve is affected?
   a. Radial
   b. Ulnar
   c. Musculocutaneous
   d. Median

153. What is a risk factor for development of cholesteatoma?
   a. Diabetes mellitus
   b. Frequent antibiotic use
   c. Loud noise exposure
   d. Chronic otitis media

154. Between what ages do epiphyseal plates typically close?
   a. 2-9
   b. 10-17
   c. 18-25
   d. 26-33

155. You are ordering a CT scan for a patient you suspect has a kidney stone. Starting at what size will the stone likely need to be removed surgically?
    a. 8 mm
    b. 5 mm
    c. 3 mm
    d. 1 mm

156. A 56-year-old man arrives in the emergency department with sudden onset of pain in his right foot. On exam, you note pale, cool skin and are unable to palpate the dorsalis pedis pulse. What is the most likely diagnosis?
    a. Acute peripheral arterial occlusion
    b. Raynaud phenomenon
    c. Deep venous thrombosis
    d. Venous insufficiency

157. All of the following are true about phenylketonuria EXCEPT:
    a. Affected children may give off a mousy body odor.
    b. It occurs most often among Jewish patients.
    c. Inheritance is autosomal recessive.
    d. It may present with seizures.

158. Which one of the following antibiotics can be ototoxic?
    a. Gentamicin
    b. Amoxicillin
    c. Levofloxacin
    d. Cefprozil

159. Which of the following medications is used to treat an acute gout attack?
    a. Methotrexate
    b. Colchicine
    c. Azathioprine
    d. Allopurinol

160. Where is the murmur of mitral regurgitation best heard on physical exam?
    a. Right lower sternal border
    b. Left upper sternal border
    c. Left fourth intercostal space
    d. Heart apex

161. A 40-year-old new patient requests to be checked for diabetes since he has a family history. His $A_{1c}$ is 6.7%. Does he meet the criteria for a diabetes diagnosis, and if so how do you treat this patient?
    a. No, advise retesting in 3 months
    b. Yes, start insulin
    c. Yes, start metformin
    d. No, advise continued diet and exercise

162. An 8-year-old boy has had 1 week of itchiness and redness on his forearms. All of the following are in your differential EXCEPT:
    a. Urticaria
    b. Atopic dermatitis
    c. Contact dermatitis
    d. Seborrheic dermatitis

163. The United States Preventive Services Task Force recommends HIV screening for which of the following patient populations?
    a. Only men and women who have had greater than 5 sexual partners
    b. All adults over the age of 18
    c. Adolescents and adults at increased risk and pregnant women
    d. Only those who are symptomatic or request to be tested

164. Which of the following lab results might you see in a patient with sarcoidosis?
    a. Elevated angiotensin-converting enzyme
    b. Decreased serum calcium
    c. Elevated white blood cells
    d. Decreased alkaline phosphatase

165. Which of the following predispose a patient to developing atrial fibrillation?
    a. Hypertension
    b. Binge drinking
    c. Hyperthyroidism
    d. All of the above

166. You are interviewing a patient with bipolar disorder who is currently having a manic episode. Which of the following best describes what you would include when documenting the mental status examination?
    a. Disheveled, guarded, looseness of associations
    b. Pressured speech, grandiose, flight of ideas
    c. Psychomotor retardation, blunted affect, suicidal ideation
    d. Tremulous, poor eye contact, obsessive ruminations

167. You have been seeing a patient with anxiety and depression who has tried many selective serotonin reuptake inhibitors (SSRIs) over the years. He would like to switch to a different medication and prefers to take something at night. One of his main symptoms is decreased appetite. Which of the following would be the best choice?
    a. Bupropion
    b. Venlafaxine
    c. Mirtazapine
    d. Citalopram

168. A 25-year-old woman arrives in the emergency department with severe headache and nausea. She is tachycardic and diaphoretic, with a blood pressure of 174/109. She has had episodes like this before and recalls a relative with a similar problem. Her plasma metanephrine is elevated. What is the most likely diagnosis?
  a. Essential hypertension
  b. Secondary aldosteronism
  c. Cushing syndrome
  d. Pheochromocytoma

169. A chalazion involves dysfunction of what structure?
  a. Sebaceous gland of Zeis
  b. Tear duct
  c. Meibomian gland
  d. Iris

170. How long should a patient with latent tuberculosis be treated with isoniazid?
  a. 2-4 weeks
  b. 1-3 months
  c. 3-6 months
  d. 6-9 months

171. A 63-year-old man reports worsening nighttime urinary frequency. On exam, you note an enlarged, rubbery prostate. Urinalysis and prostate-specific antigen (PSA) are normal. How do you treat this patient?
  a. Ampicillin
  b. Terazosin
  c. Vardenafil
  d. Oxybutynin

172. A 58-year-old woman arrives in the emergency department with palpitations and weakness. On auscultation, you note a regular rhythm. ECG shows a "sawtooth" pattern. What is the most likely diagnosis?
  a. Atrial fibrillation
  b. Wolff-Parkinson-White syndrome
  c. Atrial flutter
  d. Sinus node dysfunction

173. Oral cancer is most prevalent in which of the following patient populations?
  a. Patients who smoke and drink
  b. Patients with a history of syphilis
  c. Elderly patients because of chronic fluoride exposure
  d. Patients with skin cancer

174. A 45-year-old man arrives for routine follow-up. He reports a persistent cough for the past 2 months. On exam, you do not find signs of infection or inflammation. With further questioning, he remembers that the cough started when a new medication was added. Which medication is likely the culprit?
  a. Lisinopril
  b. Furosemide
  c. Losartan
  d. Diltiazem

175. A 21-year-old male college student arrives in the emergency department with headache and fever since yesterday. On exam, Brudzinski sign is positive. What is the mostly likely diagnosis based on this information?

a. Encephalitis

b. Subdural empyema

c. Acute transverse myelitis

d. Bacterial meningitis

176. Which of the following labs would you include in a typical workup for dementia?

a. CK

b. B12

c. AFP

d. ESR

177. Which of the following vitamins should be recommended for patients with alcohol dependence?

a. Niacin

b. Thiamine

c. Vitamin C

d. Vitamin K

178. You are doing a full body skin exam on a 45-year-old obese female patient. Across the back of her neck, you notice darkened pigmentation in the skin crease with a velvety texture. What diagnosis does this likely reflect?

a. Diabetes mellitus

b. Ulcerative colitis

c. Pyoderma gangrenosum

d. Hepatitis C

179. All of the following are true regarding iron supplementation for anemia EXCEPT:

a. The usual dose is 325 mg of ferrous sulfate given once or twice daily.

b. Parenteral iron supplementation is used for some patients.

c. Diarrhea and constipation are uncommon side effects.

d. The anemia is usually corrected within several months.

180. How is acromegaly usually treated?

a. Vasopressin

b. Recombinant growth hormone

c. Ablation of thyroid gland

d. Surgical removal or radiation of pituitary adenoma

181. A 4-year-old boy is brought in by his mother who is concerned that her son seems to be short of breath all the time. Also, he has been complaining that his head hurts and that his legs hurt when he runs. His blood pressure is elevated today. On exam, you note that his extremities are cool to the touch with diminished femoral pulses. You can hear a bruit on auscultation in the interscapular area. ECG shows left ventricular hypertrophy. What is the most likely diagnosis?

a. Coarctation of the aorta

b. Tetralogy of Fallot

c. Ventricular septal defect

d. Tricuspid atresia

182. Which of the following is true regarding barrier contraceptives?
    a. There is only one size of diaphragm that can be used over the cervix.
    b. Pregnancy rate is about 15% in a year of inconsistent condom use.
    c. Nonoxynol-10 is a type of spermicide.
    d. None of the above

183. A 55-year-old woman has pain in the area near her left cheek. On exam, you note swelling of the left side of the face near the jaw line and ear. The area is tender upon palpation, and you feel a firm lump with overlying erythema. She is febrile. What is the most likely diagnosis?
    a. Sialadenitis
    b. Temporal arteritis
    c. Ludwig angina
    d. Peritonsillar abscess

184. What cranial nerve does an acoustic neuroma affect?
    a. Third
    b. Sixth
    c. Eighth
    d. Eleventh

185. You are looking at a chest x-ray which shows small upper nodules and hilar node calcification in an "eggshell" pattern. What does this likely suggest?
    a. Asbestosis
    b. Mediastinitis
    c. Goodpasture syndrome
    d. Silicosis

186. All of the following are used in the treatment of osteoarthritis EXCEPT:
    a. Oral steroids
    b. Acetaminophen
    c. NSAIDs
    d. Celecoxib

187. A 40-year-old man has progressive difficulty swallowing and pain behind the sternum. He says that he also tends to regurgitate some of his food in the nighttime. Barium x-ray shows absence of progressive esophageal contractions with a narrow lower segment. What is most likely diagnosis?
    a. Hiatal hernia
    b. GERD
    c. Achalasia
    d. Mallory-Weiss syndrome

188. A 52-year-old man arrives after a fall he sustained several days ago. He is now having severe hip pain with walking along with limited motion. On exam, you hear a click when externally rotating the hip. X-ray shows a "crescent sign." He is diagnosed with a hip fracture, but what else is complicating his presentation?
    a. Osteoporosis
    b. Paget disease of bone
    c. Osteomyelitis
    d. Avascular necrosis

189. You are monitoring a patient with atrial fibrillation who has been taking warfarin. He had laboratory tests done earlier today, and his international normalized ratio (INR) was at 3.9. What do you need to do?
    a. Increase the dose
    b. Decrease the dose
    c. Keep dose the same
    d. Discontinue medication

190. Which of the following patient populations has the highest rate of death by suicide?
    a. Elderly males
    b. Adolescent males
    c. Adolescent females
    d. Pregnant women

191. You are counseling a patient about the benefits of smoking cessation. Which of the following could you include in your discussion of conditions that are associated with smoking?
    a. Bladder carcinoma
    b. Nephrolithiasis
    c. Polycystic kidney disease
    d. Interstitial cystitis

192. What is the physiology behind urticaria?
    a. Impaired venous drainage
    b. Sebaceous duct obstruction
    c. Histamine release
    d. Spread of bacterial infection

193. You are seeing a 45-year-old male patient for the second time. The average of his two blood pressure readings in office is 135/78. How would you classify this?
    a. Normal
    b. Prehypertension
    c. Stage 1 hypertension
    d. Stage 2 hypertension

194. A blood test for CA-125 may be ordered for a patient if which condition is suspected?
    a. Ovarian cancer
    b. Incompetent cervix
    c. Uterine prolapse
    d. Primary amenorrhea

195. What medication is typically prescribed to patients for recurrent Raynaud phenomenon?
    a. Furosemide
    b. Prednisone
    c. Gabapentin
    d. Nifedipine

196. You are seeing a patient who takes sulfasalazine for ulcerative colitis. What is a potential side effect of this medication?
    a. Pancreatitis
    b. Oligospermia
    c. Blindness
    d. Priapism

197. In a 24-hour period, how many milligrams of excreted albumin in urine is considered to be macroalbuminuria?
    a. > 300
    b. > 200
    c. > 100
    d. > 50

198. Which of the following is an indication for open reduction and internal fixation (ORIF) surgery?
    a. Hip fracture
    b. Displaced fracture of both radius and ulna
    c. Displaced intra-articular fracture of the knee
    d. All of the above

199. A 39-year-old man has left elbow pain that has been present for 2 weeks. He cannot recall a specific injury. On exam, you note bogginess around the elbow and pain elicited with elbow flexion. There is no erythema. What is the most likely diagnosis?
    a. Gout
    b. Biceps tendon rupture
    c. Olecranon bursitis
    d. Osteoarthritis

200. You order an echocardiogram on a patient who has congestive heart failure. What would you expect his ejection fraction to be?
    a. 80%
    b. 65%
    c. 55%
    d. 40%

201. Which of the following is NOT usually recommended in the management of fibrocystic changes of the breasts?
    a. Increase caffeine intake
    b. Restrict foods containing methylxanthine
    c. Use mild diuretics intermittently
    d. Take danazol regularly

202. You are reading through a chart and notice "hemiballismus" documented in the neurological section of the physical exam. What does this refer to?
    a. Slowness of movements and reflexes
    b. Involuntary violent flinging movements of the extremities
    c. Dance-like irregular movements
    d. Rhythmic limb movements

203. What is contained in the hormonal intrauterine device?
   a. Ethinyl estradiol
   b. Mestranol
   c. Levonorgestrel
   d. Estradiol valerate

204. Which imaging modality is most often used for detecting the presence of kidney stones?
   a. MRI
   b. Cystoscopy
   c. KUB
   d. Ultrasound

205. A 32-year-old woman has had progressive redness and swelling for the past week in the area under her right eye close to the side of her nose. The area is tender to palpation. Tearing and discharge are present. Vision is intact. What is the most likely diagnosis?
   a. Dacryocystitis
   b. Orbital cellulitis
   c. Pinguecula
   d. Chalazion

206. A 27-year-old woman has had persistent fever after returning from a trip to Africa. *Plasmodium ovale* is seen in the peripheral blood smear. How can this patient be treated?
   a. Chloroquine
   b. Metronidazole
   c. Sulfadiazine
   d. Albendazole

207. What would you expect to find while performing a physical examination of a patient with only left-sided heart failure?
   a. Jugular venous distention
   b. Hepatomegaly
   c. Lung crackles
   d. Pedal edema

208. A 2-year-old boy arrives in your office in October with a barking cough present for the past 3 days. On exam, you note retractions and hear a high-pitched sound with inspiration. There is no drooling or sputum production, and you do not notice pharyngeal swelling. What do you suspect?
   a. Croup
   b. Bronchiectasis
   c. Acute bronchitis
   d. Peritonsillar abscess

209. All of the following are indications for biosynthetic valve replacement EXCEPT:
   a. Women who wish to become pregnant
   b. Younger than 65 years
   c. Contraindication for anticoagulation
   d. Endocarditis

210. Approximately how many women will experience domestic violence in their lifetime?
a. 5%
b. 15%
c. 25%
d. 40%

211. A patient has extreme thirst and excessive urination. Urine is diluted with no glucose present. Serum blood glucose is normal, although sodium level is elevated. What is the most likely diagnosis based on this information?
a. Diabetes insipidus
b. Urinary tract infection
c. Diabetes mellitus
d. Acute renal failure

212. Which of the following results from an arterial blood gas test would suggest respiratory acidosis?
a. pH of 7.5
b. Decreased $PaCO_2$
c. pH of 7.4
d. Increased $PaCO_2$

213. You are looking at an x-ray of a child's fractured radius. Your supervising physician says it is a Salter-Harris type II fracture. What bone structures does this fracture effect?
a. Physis, metaphysis, and epiphysis
b. Physis and epiphysis
c. Physis and metaphysis
d. Physis only

214. A 30-year-old man has rectal pain and reports bright red blood on the tissue paper after defecation. Upon inspection, you see a small area of swelling and erythema near the rectum. What prescription will provide some relief for this patient?
a. Mesalamine
b. Loperamide
c. Rifaximin
d. Docusate

215. Metoprolol is used to treat which of the following?
a. Severe bradycardia
b. Hypertension
c. Third-degree AV block
d. All of the above

216. A 56-year-old man with a history of smoking and congestive heart failure has worsening shortness of breath. On exam, you note dullness to percussion and decreased breath sounds on the side of the left lung. What is likely going on here?
a. Pleural effusion
b. Acute bronchitis
c. Pneumothorax
d. Emphysema

217. Which of the following is NOT associated with a diagnosis of macular degeneration?
    a. Presence of drusen
    b. Loss of peripheral vision
    c. Development of scotomas
    d. Deteriorating vision in elderly patients

218. You are asking a new 32-year-old male patient about his medical and surgical history. He says that he had previously sustained a rotator cuff injury. Which one of the following muscles might have been affected?
    a. Deltoid
    b. Teres minor
    c. Rhomboideus major
    d. Teres major

219. A 45-year-old woman arrives in the emergency department with a blood pressure of 207/134. A family member says that she has not been taking any of her medications for the past few weeks. The patient is found to be confused with elevated creatinine. How do you best treat this patient?
    a. IV nicardipine
    b. Oral nitroglycerin
    c. IV furosemide
    d. Oral clonidine

220. Which of the following would you NOT expect when performing a physical examination of a patient with myasthenia gravis?
    a. Diplopia
    b. Ptosis
    c. Muscle weakness
    d. Decreased deep tendon reflexes

221. A 26-year-old man arrives in the emergency department with periumbilical pain that has been present for the past 3 hours. On exam, you note abdominal guarding and tenderness at McBurney point. What is your next step?
    a. Order a right upper quadrant (RUQ) ultrasound
    b. Call surgery
    c. Discharge with pain medications
    d. Advise a high-fiber diet

222. A 22-year-old man has low-grade flank pain. He is hypertensive, and urinalysis shows blood and protein. CT shows bilateral enlarged kidneys with multiple fluid-filled spaces. What is the most likely diagnosis?
    a. Urinary tract infection
    b. Nephrolithiasis
    c. Polycystic kidney disease
    d. Pyelonephritis

223. Which medication is most suitable for treating lichen simplex chronicus?
    a. Tretinoin
    b. Nystatin
    c. Neomycin
    d. Triamcinolone

224. You are reviewing a patient's lymph node biopsy results which reveal Reed-Sternberg cells. What are these cells associated with?
    a. Burkitt lymphoma
    b. Multiple myeloma
    c. Hodgkin lymphoma
    d. Acute lymphoblastic leukemia

225. What is the mechanism of action for fluvoxamine?
    a. Serotonin 5-HT receptor partial agonist
    b. Serotonin-norepinephrine reuptake inhibitor
    c. Norepinephrine-dopamine reuptake inhibitor
    d. Selective serotonin reuptake inhibitor

226. A 12-year-old girl arrives in the emergency department with nausea, vomiting, and abdominal pain. She is hypotensive and tachycardic. Glucose and ketones are present in the urine. What does this patient likely have?
    a. Addison disease
    b. Type I diabetes mellitus
    c. Multiple endocrine neoplasia
    d. Type II diabetes mellitus

227. What is torsades de pointes?
    a. Polymorphic ventricular tachycardia associated with long QT syndrome
    b. Partial or complete interruption of impulse conduction in a bundle branch
    c. Reentrant supraventricular tachycardia triggered by an atrial premature beat
    d. Rapid regular atrial rhythm due to a reentrant circuit

228. A 34-year-old generally healthy man has had cough, shortness of breath, pleuritic chest pain, and malaise for the past 3 days. He is febrile, and crackles are heard with lung auscultation. Chest x-ray shows multilobar infiltrates. What is the most likely causative organism?
    a. Adenovirus
    b. *Histoplasma capsulatum*
    c. *Streptococcus pneumoniae*
    d. Respiratory syncytial virus

229. Epidemiologically, which one of the following patients would be the most likely to be diagnosed with sarcoidosis?
    a. 32-year-old African-American woman
    b. 16-year-old Asian male adolescent
    c. 63-year-old Caucasian woman
    d. 41-year-old Hispanic man

230. A growing pituitary adenoma can compress which of the following structures?
    a. Superior cerebellar peduncle
    b. Optic chiasm
    c. Pineal body
    d. Amygdala

231. Which of the following medications does NOT typically have gastrointestinal side effects?
    a. Citalopram
    b. Metformin
    c. Naproxen
    d. Albuterol

232. A 70-year-old man who recently had abdominal surgery has a swollen, painful, erythematous left lower leg. He does not recall any trauma to the leg. D-dimer is positive. When doing your physical examination, what would help support your suspected diagnosis?
    a. Murphy sign
    b. Homan sign
    c. Waddell sign
    d. Tinel sign

233. According to the latest guidelines from the American Congress of Obstetricians and Gynecologists, at what age should women start having annual mammograms?
    a. 55
    b. 30
    c. 50
    d. 40

234. How can primary pulmonary hypertension be treated?
    a. Prostaglandins
    b. Norepinephrine
    c. Beta-agonists
    d. Antidiuretic hormone

235. A 67-year-old woman has urinary symptoms of urgency and frequency for the past year, to the point where she leaks urine. Her urinalysis is negative for infection. Which muscle is over-active in this case?
    a. External sphincter
    b. Detrusor
    c. Internal sphincter
    d. Trigone

236. A 50-year-old man with hypertension arrives for routine follow-up. He reports that he had a 5-minute episode last week where his vision went black in one eye. On today's exam, you do not find any visual deficits. What likely happened to this patient?
    a. Subarachnoid hemorrhage
    b. Central retinal artery occlusion
    c. Transient ischemic attack
    d. Optic neuritis

237. All of the following are associated with a diagnosis of rheumatoid arthritis EXCEPT:
    a. Radial deviation of the fingers
    b. Boutonniere deformity
    c. Keratoconjunctivitis sicca
    d. Anti-CCP

238. A 40-year-old man has right ankle pain that started suddenly when he was running earlier in the day. When doing your physical examination, you find that the Thompson test is positive. What does this signify?
    a. Ankle sprain
    b. Achilles tendon rupture
    c. Talus fracture
    d. Gastrocnemius tear

239. You have been treating a 54-year-old male patient with simvastatin for hyperlipidemia. Recent lab results show that his LDL and HDL are at goal, but his triglycerides are still very elevated. What medication could you add to target this?
    a. Colestipol
    b. Fenofibrate
    c. Cholestyramine
    d. Rosuvastatin

240. A 30-year-old woman has fever and neck pain that started several days ago. She says that she had just been getting over an upper respiratory tract infection. On exam, you note that her thyroid gland is tender to palpation and enlarged. Her free $T_4$ is elevated, and TSH is decreased. Radioactive iodine uptake is decreased. How do you treat this patient?
    a. NSAIDs
    b. Levothyroxine
    c. Thyroidectomy
    d. Radioiodine

241. Which of the following arteries provides blood supply to the heart itself?
    a. Left circumflex
    b. Right marginal
    c. Left anterior descending
    d. All of the above

242. What is a Schilling test used for?
    a. Detecting the presence of antibodies on the surface of RBCs
    b. Testing for iron deficiency
    c. Determining whether vitamin B12 is being absorbed normally
    d. Measuring different types of hemoglobin in the blood

243. A 17-year-old male adolescent has had fever, abdominal pain, and nausea for 4 days. He notes that he had gone swimming in a local pond several weeks prior. He is not sexually active. On exam, he is noted to have jaundice of the eyes. His ALT is elevated. What is the most likely diagnosis?
    a. Hepatitis A
    b. Hepatitis B
    c. Hepatitis C
    d. Hepatitis D

244. Which of the following is a risk factor for placenta previa?
    a. Gestational diabetes
    b. Use of oxytocin
    c. Previous cesarean sections
    d. Cervical cancer

245. You have been treating patient with refractory depression who would like to try electroconvulsive therapy. What is a potential well-documented effect of the procedure that he should be aware of?
    a. Development of obstructive sleep apnea
    b. Increased risk of brain cancer
    c. Cognitive and memory dysfunction
    d. Chronic diarrhea

246. A 27-year-old woman has had left eye redness for the past 3 days. On exam, you note conjunctival erythema and a yellowish discharge from the eye with crusting. Vision is intact, and nasal passages are clear. How do you treat this patient?
    a. Moxifloxacin
    b. Betadine
    c. Diphenhydramine
    d. Olopatadine

247. At what age is the first dose of the DTaP vaccine recommended?
    a. 1 month
    b. 2 months
    c. 6 months
    d. 1 year

248. What is the basic pathophysiology of shock?
    a. Low blood pressure
    b. Excess norepinephrine
    c. Inadequate cellular oxygen supply
    d. Retention of fluids

249. At what gestational age are maternal serum genetic screening tests usually offered to pregnant women?
    a. 15-20 weeks
    b. 21-24 weeks
    c. 24-28 weeks
    d. 28-32 weeks

250. You are performing CPR and notice that the chest is not rising whenever you do rescue breaths. You ensure that the head and neck are in the right position, but you are still not seeing chest movement. What is a possible reason for this?
    a. Drug overdose
    b. Cardiac arrest
    c. Pulmonary hemorrhage
    d. Foreign body aspiration

251. All of the following medications are nephrotoxic EXCEPT:
    a. Gentamicin
    b. Amphotericin B
    c. Mycophenolate
    d. Penicillin

252. A 50-year-old man with a history of rheumatic fever arrives for follow-up. Upon exam, you hear a holosystolic murmur at the heart apex. What does this signify?
    a. Aortic regurgitation
    b. Mitral stenosis
    c. Aortic stenosis
    d. Mitral regurgitation

253. You are seeing a patient who was recently diagnosed with exocrine pancreatic cancer. He has been told that surgery is not an option. You are having a discussion about end-of-life care, and he wants to know what his 5-year survival rate is. What is the approximation you tell him?
    a. 5%
    b. 25%
    c. 40%
    d. 65%

254. Which of the following is a correct pairing?
    a. Cranial nerve I - optic
    b. Cranial nerve IV - trigeminal
    c. Cranial nerve VIII - vestibulocochlear
    d. All of the above

255. You are ordering fasting labs for a patient as part of routine follow-up. What is the range for diagnosis of impaired fasting glucose according to the American Diabetes Association?
    a. < 100 mg/dL
    b. 100-125 mg/dL
    c. 126-140 mg/dL
    d. > 140 mg/dL

256. A 32-year-old male patient has been in a cast for a tibial fracture. Today he presents with excruciating pain in the anterior leg. On exam, the leg is pale and pulses are weak. His report of pain seems to be out of proportion to what is found on physical exam. What is the most likely diagnosis?
    a. Peripheral arterial disease
    b. Deep venous thrombosis
    c. Fibula fracture
    d. Compartment syndrome

257. All of the following are medications used to treatment human immunodeficiency virus EXCEPT:
    a. Ribavirin
    b. Abacavir
    c. Efavirenz
    d. Ritonavir

258. Approximately what percentage of the United States population has asthma?
    a. 2%
    b. 8%
    c. 15%
    d. 31%

259. When performing a physical examination, what can you ask the patient to do in order for the murmur of aortic stenosis to become intensified?
   a. Squat
   b. Lean backwards
   c. "Bear down" as if having a bowel movement
   d. Clench fists

260. A 34-year-old woman has the complaint of "heartburn," which she says is worse at night and after eating certain foods. How could you treat this patient?
   a. Polyethylene glycol
   b. Lipase
   c. Ondansetron
   d. Omeprazole

261. What is the one of the risks of amniocentesis?
   a. Gestational diabetes
   b. Preeclampsia
   c. Preterm labor
   d. Placenta previa

262. You are seeing a 58-year-old male patient with schizoaffective disorder for follow-up. During the interview, you notice that he is continually smacking his lips and sometimes sticking his tongue out. He does not seem to be aware of these movements or bothered by them. What can you likely attribute these movements to?
   a. Increased anxiety
   b. Side effect from medication
   c. Habit present since childhood
   d. Recently finished eating

263. A 20-year-old man had sudden onset of right ear pain when he woke up. On otoscopic exam, you note that there is actually a small live insect in the ear canal. Which medication should you use prior to attempting removal of the insect?
   a. Lidocaine
   b. Hydrocortisone
   c. Ciprofloxacin
   d. Triamcinolone

264. A 45-year-old woman has had worsening bilateral leg weakness for the past several months. She says that her legs get tired easily when walking or going up stairs. On exam, her thigh muscles are mildly tender and atrophied. You do not notice any rashes. You run a series of tests and find that CK is elevated. Muscle biopsy shows chronic inflammation and degeneration. What is the most likely diagnosis?
   a. Dermatomyositis
   b. Guillain-Barré syndrome
   c. Polymyositis
   d. Systemic lupus erythematosus

265. Which of the following medications is used for cigarette smoking cessation?
   a. Disulfiram
   b. Varenicline
   c. Buprenorphine
   d. Acamprosate

266. All of the following are sections of the stomach EXCEPT:
   a. Cardia
   b. Fundus
   c. Body
   d. Gastrus

267. A 67-year-old obese man arrives for routine follow-up. He does not have any specific complaints today. As you are performing an abdominal exam, you note a small bulge around the umbilicus that seems to reduce in size with pressure. What is the likely problem?
   a. Hernia
   b. Abscess
   c. Tumor
   b. Cyst

268. How can you treat acute bronchiolitis?
   a. Antibiotics
   b. Corticosteroids
   c. Oxygen
   d. Aspirin

269. What is a potential complication of thyroidectomy?
   a. Hyperthyroidism
   b. Hoarseness
   c. Hyperparathyroidism
   d. Loss of taste

270. Approximately how many weeks does it take after egg fertilization for a urine pregnancy test to have a positive result?
   a. 7-8
   b. 5-6
   c. 3-4
   d. 1-2

271. A 54-year-old obese male patient with hypertension arrives for routine follow-up. He reports that he is not sleeping well at night and that he feels tired during the day. His wife says that he snores loudly. What is the next best step in management of this patient?
   a. Prescribe zolpidem for insomnia
   b. Encourage daytime naps
   c. Order a sleep study
   d. Prescribe modafinil to improve wakefulness

272. You are reviewing the chart of a patient that has been receiving psychiatric treatment for years; the patient has requested to switch providers for the third time. You note a history of childhood abuse, low distress tolerance, substance abuse, and multiple suicide attempts. Which personality disorder is this patient likely diagnosed with?
    a. Paranoid
    b. Antisocial
    c. Avoidant
    d. Borderline

273. An 18-year-old generally healthy woman reports intermittent episodes where she feels like her heart is beating very fast. She cannot pinpoint any specific triggers but says this has been going on for months. She does not have a history of anxiety. On exam, you do not hear any murmurs. Her ECG is normal today. What is the best next step?
    a. Have her return in 6 months
    b. Order an echocardiogram
    c. Have her undergo Holter monitoring
    d. Order a stress test

274. All of the following are used to treat osteoporosis EXCEPT:
    a. Risedronate
    b. Raloxifene
    c. Zoledronic acid
    d. Carisoprodol

275. Name the correct order of the connective tissue membranes surrounding the spinal cord, starting from the spinal cord and going outwards.
    a. Pia mater, subarachnoid space, arachnoid mater, dura mater
    b. Subarachnoid space, arachnoid mater, pia mater, dura mater
    c. Pia mater, dura mater, subarachnoid space, arachnoid mater
    d. Dura mater, subarachnoid space, arachnoid mater, pia mater

276. All of the following are true regarding the management of folate deficiency EXCEPT:
    a. Encourage dietary inclusion of plant foods and meats.
    b. Prescribe folic acid as a daily supplement.
    c. Advise patient that deficiency in pregnancy can lead to neural tube defects.
    d. Instruct patient to overcook food so that folate is preserved.

277. What is the function of the greater omentum in the abdominal cavity?
    a. Connects the left kidney to the spleen
    b. Walls off inflammation
    c. Absorbs nutrients
    d. All of the above

278. All of the following are located in the hilum within the root of each lung EXCEPT:
    a. Two pulmonary veins
    b. Main bronchus
    c. Two pulmonary arteries
    d. Nerves

279. A 32-year-old woman has eye redness and tearing. Vision is decreased. You do fluorescein dye staining and see dendritic corneal lesions. What does this signify?
   a. Bacterial conjunctivitis
   b. Herpes keratitis
   c. Iritis
   d. Optic neuritis

280. A 45-year-old woman is a new patient. She has not been to a doctor in several years but does not have any specific complaints today. During your physical exam, you notice that her right breast has an area that appears like the texture of an orange peel. Why is this concerning?
   a. Fibrocystic changes
   b. Breast cancer
   c. Mastitis
   d. Herpes zoster

281. A 50-year-old man with lupus has worsening peripheral edema and a report of frothy urine. The 24-hour urine collection shows protein loss of 4.2 grams. What is the most likely diagnosis?
   a. Renal artery occlusion
   b. Acute tubular necrosis
   c. Acute renal failure
   d. Nephrotic syndrome

282. How can a large pleural effusion be treated if it is resulting in pulmonary dysfunction?
   a. Paracentesis
   b. Physiotherapy
   c. Thoracentesis
   d. Nebulizer

283. Which of the following is a risk factor for development of endometrial cancer?
   a. Obesity
   b. Cigarette smoking
   c. HPV infection
   d. Unopposed progesterone

284. All of the following conditions would show an obstructive pattern on pulmonary function tests EXCEPT:
   a. Asthma
   b. Chronic bronchitis
   c. Chest wall disease
   d. Emphysema

285. A 46-year-old man with a history of *H. pylori* infection arrives for follow-up of dyspepsia. Now he says that he feels full even if he has not eaten much. He is found to be anemic with loss of weight and lymphadenopathy. What is the most likely diagnosis?
   a. Pancreatic cancer
   b. Colon cancer
   c. Liver cancer
   d. Stomach cancer

286. What is incised when performing a midline episiotomy?
    a. External urethral sphincter
    b. Perineal body
    c. Inferior pubic ligament
    d. Rectal ampulla

287. Which of the following is an indication for ordering an upper GI endoscopy?
    a. Banding of varices
    b. Hematochezia
    c. Sore throat
    d. Evaluation of the ileum

288. What is the mechanism of action for montelukast?
    a. Beta-2 agonist
    b. Antihistamine
    c. Leukotriene receptor antagonist
    d. Anticholinergic

289. When performing a physical examination of the lungs, what can a finding of increased tactile fremitus signify?
    a. Hyperinflation
    b. Consolidation
    c. Emphysema
    d. Bronchial obstruction

290. A 12-year-old girl has persistent fever and loss of weight. On exam, you note pale skin, petechiae, hepatosplenomegaly, and enlarged lymph nodes. WBC is extremely elevated with blast cells seen in peripheral smear. What is the most likely diagnosis?
    a. Chronic lymphocytic leukemia
    b. Acute myelogenous leukemia
    c. Chronic myelogenous leukemia
    d. Acute lymphoblastic leukemia

291. A mother brings in her 6-year-old son with the complaint that he does not seem to be listening at school or at home. She says that he jumps from thing to thing and makes careless mistakes on schoolwork. During the appointment, he is fidgety, has a hard time staying seated, and interrupts often. How can this condition be treated?
    a. Benzodiazepines
    b. Mood stabilizers
    c. Stimulants
    d. Antipsychotics

292. You are about to perform a lumbar puncture on a patient with suspected meningitis. Between which vertebral levels should you insert the needle?
    a. L3 and L4
    b. L1 and L2
    c. S1 and S2
    d. S3 and S4

293. A 45-year-old woman has a painless lump in her neck. On exam, you note a thyroid nodule. Biopsy reveals thyroid cancer. What is the most likely type?
    a. Follicular
    b. Papillary
    c. Medullary
    d. Anaplastic

294. A 72-year-old woman arrives for routine follow-up. You notice that her height has actually decreased over the past few years. On exam, the mid to upper part of her back has a "hump" deformity. What does this patient have?
    a. Scoliosis
    b. Lordosis
    c. Swayback
    d. Kyphosis

295. Which medication can be used to treat moderate pulmonary cryptococcosis in an immunocompromised patient?
    a. Fluconazole
    b. Nystatin
    c. Terbinafine
    d. Selenium

296. What does ocular tonometry evaluate for?
    a. Glaucoma
    b. Strabismus
    c. Cataract
    d. Retinoblastoma

297. A 24-year-old woman arrives in the emergency department. She reports having food poisoning and says that she has been vomiting for the past 3 days, but today she noticed blood in her vomit. Upper endoscopy shows a superficial tear in the esophagus but no active bleeding. How do you treat this patient?
    a. Prescribe omeprazole
    b. No other intervention needed at this time
    c. Order a barium esophagography
    d. Laparotomy

298. What is the approximate therapeutic range for lithium?
    a. 5.2–5.8 mEq/L
    b. 3.5–4.5 mEq/L
    c. 1.5–3.0 mEq/L
    d. 0.6–1.2 mEq/L

299. A 21-year-old man has discharge from his penis and painful urination. You do a urethral swab wet mount and see flagellated pear-shaped organisms under the microscope. What does this signify?
    a. Chlamydia
    b. Trichomoniasis
    c. Giardiasis
    d. Gonorrhea

300. You are examining a patient who has yellowing of the eyes, an enlarged spleen, spider angiomas, and a rounded firm abdomen with enlarged veins. What does this patient likely have?
    a. Cirrhosis
    b. Hepatitis A
    c. Cholecystitis
    d. HIV

# Answers and Explanations

**1. B: Atorvastatin.** This medication is an HMG-CoA reductase inhibitor and is used to treat hypercholesterolemia. Myalgias are a common side effect. More rarely, the statin medications can cause rhabdomyolysis, which may present with renal dysfunction. Niacin is also a medication used to manage cholesterol, but flushing is more common side effect.

**2. D: Not order a PSA test since the harm outweighs the benefit of screening.** The USPSTF recommends against PSA-based screening for prostate cancer. African Americans and those with a family history of prostate cancer are at a higher risk of developing prostate cancer. There are other organizations that do recommend screening for prostate cancer with the PSA test.

**3. C: Advise her that the condition will likely resolve on its own.** Based on the information given, this patient likely has a subconjunctival hemorrhage. They are usually caused by coughing, sneezing, or straining. They generally clear up on their own in a couple of weeks.

**4. A: Buspirone.** Buspirone is an anti-anxiety medication that is taken daily to reduce symptoms of generalized anxiety. Clonazepam is in the benzodiazepine class of medications and is usually used on an as-needed, short-term basis. It is generally avoided in patients with a history of substance dependence because of its potential for abuse. While bupropion and doxepin may also relieve anxiety symptoms, they are primarily used to treat depression.

**5. C: Not contagious since this is an autoimmune condition.** The condition described is lichen planus, which is thought to be an autoimmune condition that is T cell-mediated. It is usually characterized by the "Ps"—pruritic, polygonal, planar, purple, papules/plaques. Lesions can also occur on the oral mucosa. A biopsy can confirm the diagnosis, and it is treated with steroids.

**6. B: Crescendo-decrescendo ejection murmur.** Aortic stenosis is a narrowing of the aortic valve between the left ventricle and the aorta. The murmur is heard when blood is flowing from the heart to the rest of the body. Aortic regurgitation is when blood is flowing in the wrong direction from the aorta back into the left ventricle, and it can sound high-pitched. A holosystolic murmur is heard with mitral regurgitation when blood is flowing in the wrong direction from the left ventricle to the left atrium. Mitral stenosis is a narrowing of the valve between the left atrium and left ventricle, and the rumbling murmur would occur during diastole.

**7. C: Atrial fibrillation.** This arrhythmia is caused by disorganized atrial activity. The patient has risks factors such as advanced age and underlying heart problems. A patient with a myocardial infarction may present with shortness of breath, along with other symptoms like chest pain; however, the heart rhythm is not characteristically irregularly irregular. Pericardial effusion would present with diminished heart sounds due to the fluid surrounding the heart. Patients with aortic stenosis may have normal ECGs or ventricular hypertrophy.

**8. C: Irritable bowel syndrome.** IBS is a condition characterized by diarrhea and/or constipation. It has no clear cause but is common, especially in younger patients. Celiac disease is a condition in which the body reacts to the ingestion of gluten (which includes wheat), so this patient would have likely seen a reduction in her symptoms with changes in her diet. Crohn disease and ulcerative colitis are inflammatory bowel diseases that would likely show evidence of lesions on the studies performed.

9. D: Bone marrow biopsy. Anemia can be acute or chronic. In women of childbearing age, anemia can be due to iron-deficiency and treated with supplementation and diet changes. A CBC can help determine the cause of anemia, along with additional iron studies that may be necessary. It is important to evaluate for active bleeding and clinical stability. Stool studies can show occult bleeding from the GI tract. A bone marrow biopsy may be indicated at some point, but it is not a first step due to its invasiveness.

10. A: Toxoplasmosis. This is an infection that can present with a range of symptoms, but the disease occurs mostly in immunocompromised patients. The other answer choices can also occur in AIDS patients. Kaposi sarcoma usually presents as cutaneous lesions. *Pneumocystis jiroveci* and *Mycobacterium avium* complex infections usually involve the lungs.

11. B: Prescribe topical antibiotics and steroids. Otitis externa is an infection of the ear canal and is diagnosed by history and inspection. It is often called "swimmer's ear." It can be caused by bacteria or fungi. Treatment is with topical antibiotics and steroids. A cotton wick may also be used. Oral antibiotics may be necessary when cellulitis is present.

12. D: All of the above. The condition described is cryptorchidism, which is the failure of one or both testes to descend into the scrotum. It is more common in preterm infants. In most cases, the testis will spontaneously descend, but otherwise surgery should be done around the age of 6 months.

13. C: Scaphoid. This wrist bone is located on the radial side, whereas the other wrist bones listed are more medial. Scaphoid fractures usually occur with hyperextension, as seen during a fall. A common complication is avascular necrosis. Initial x-rays may be normal and require MRI, or suspected scaphoid fractures can be treated with a thumb spica splint.

14. C: LFTs and lipid panel. The epidemic of childhood obesity is due to multiple factors including genetics, diseases, medications, activity level, and diet/nutrition. The rate of childhood obesity is highest between ages 10 and 11 years. A fasting lipid profile is recommended for children between the ages of 2 and 10 years with a family history of dyslipidemia, cardiovascular disease, hypertension, diabetes, and obesity. Oral glucose tolerance testing should begin at age 10 for any child at increased risk for metabolic syndrome. For children with a body mass index (BMI) in the 95th percentile or higher, they should have LFTs, fasting glucose, and insulin and lipid profiles.

15. D: Substantia nigra. The patient described has Parkinson disease, which is a degenerative CNS disorder in which dopamine-producing cells in the substantia nigra are lost. The cause of this cell death is unknown. The substantia nigra is part of the midbrain. High levels of melanin in the dopaminergic cells give them a darker appearance. Levodopa is used as treatment in Parkinson disease because it is a metabolic precursor to dopamine.

16. A: Advise him to be cautious because this condition can spread with or without active lesions. Based on the information given, this patient has herpes simplex virus (HSV). Oral lesions are usually caused by HSV type 1, and virus shedding can occur with close contact. Diagnosis is often clinical but a Tzanck smear can confirm diagnosis. The duration of an eruption can be decreased with antivirals. HSV can appear similar to the herpes zoster virus; however, this condition is usually found in a dermatomal pattern and more painful.

17. B: Working in a chemical factory. This would not necessarily increase someone's risk of acquiring tuberculosis (TB). This mycobacterium infection is spread by inhalation, and is enhanced by

- 152 -

overcrowding or close contact. Other risk factors for acquiring TB include being homeless, being in jail or prison, living in an institution, and having HIV.

18. D: Glyburide. This medication is a sulfonylurea drug, which is an insulin secretagogue. Acarbose works by inhibiting intestinal enzymes so that carbohydrates are digested more slowly. Metformin is a biguanide that acts as an insulin sensitizer by decreasing hepatic glucose production. Pioglitazone falls under the thiazolidinedione class, which decreases peripheral insulin resistance.

19. C: Giant cell arteritis. Giant cell arteritis is also known as temporal arteritis and is a chronic inflammatory disease. It usually occurs in older adults and may present with symptoms such as headache, changes in vision, pain in the temple area, fever, and fatigue. An elevated ESR or CRP can increase suspicion for the diagnosis, which can then be verified through biopsy. It is treated with prednisone. Polymyalgia rheumatica is a condition that is associated with giant cell arteritis; it may present with similar symptoms and also include elevated ESR, but biopsy is normal.

20. A: Tetralogy of Fallot. This congenital heart condition consists of four abnormalities: ventricular septal defect, right ventricular outflow obstruction, right ventricular hypertrophy, and an overriding aorta. Although medications can be given to help with cyanotic spells, definitive treatment of the condition is by surgery.

21. D: Intussusception. This condition is when part of the intestine "telescopes" into another part. It usually occurs between 3 months and 3 years of age. It can lead to bowel obstruction or ischemia if not treated. Pyloric stenosis usually presents with projectile vomiting. Meconium ileus and necrotizing enterocolitis occur in neonates.

22. D: Meniscus tear. This type of injury would elicit a positive McMurray test, in which the examiner can feel a "click" in the knee while extending and rotating the leg. Anterior cruciate ligament (ACL) and lateral collateral ligament (LCL) tears are possible given the mechanism of injury in this patient, but these injuries alone would not have a positive McMurray test. An ACL tear would have a positive Lachman test, which is where anterior motion can be felt while pulling upwards on the tibia compared with the femur.

23. C: Elevated pressure, neutrophils > 2000/mcL, glucose < 40 mg/dL, protein > 100 mg/dL. In adults, bacterial meningitis is usually caused by pneumococci. The bacteria draw neutrophils into the CSF space. Pressure is increased because of release of metabolites that damage cell membranes. Glucose is usually lower because it is being consumed by bacteria and neutrophils.

24. A: Sick sinus syndrome, also known as sinus node dysfunction, refers to any condition where the atrial rate is abnormal. Patients may present with weakness, dizziness, or palpitations. Dropped P waves can trigger escape beats from other parts of the heart. Treatment is by pacemaker. Wandering atrial pacemaker, also known as multifocal atrial rhythm, would show varied P waves. Wolff-Parkinson-White syndrome would show short PR intervals and delta waves.

25. C: Hydrochlorothiazide. This man is considered to have stage 1 hypertension, which is systolic between 140-159 mm Hg or diastolic between 90-99 mm Hg. Thiazide-type diuretics are recommended initially for most patients. Patients with stage 2 hypertension will likely require two medications for blood pressure control. In patients with certain medical problems, other drugs are initially recommended. For example, an ACE inhibitor or angiotensin receptor blocker would be advised instead for a patient with chronic kidney disease.

26. A: Inferior rectus. A blowout fracture involves the bones surrounding the eye, usually caused by blunt trauma. Inferior fractures are the most common. The inferior rectus muscle can become entrapped, causing limited motion of the eye and changes in vision. The "teardrop sign" is the orbital contents and muscle protruding into the sinus cavity.

27. C: Permethrin cream applied to the whole body. The patient described has scabies, which is caused by the mite *Sarcoptes scabiei*. The mites burrow in the skin and cause severe itching. It is easily transmitted through contact. Diagnosis is usually based on history and observation but can also be confirmed through skin scrapings. The permethrin cream is applied all over and washed off after several hours. Treatment should be repeated in 1 week, and all personal items should be washed.

28. A: 9 years old with distal radius fracture. This is a common injury usually due to falling on an outstretched hand. For the other x-rays listed, the forces involved to break those bones are much more than would be expected in a simple childhood accident.

29. C: Testicular torsion. This condition occurs mostly in teenagers and can be spontaneous or as a result of trauma. It is considered an emergency because of the strangulation of blood supply. Ischemia and necrosis will occur if not promptly treated. A varicocele is not necessarily painful and may feel like a "bag of worms" on exam because of enlarged veins in the scrotum. Testicular cancer would not present with such acute pain. Hydroceles are painless collections of fluid in the scrotum.

30. D: Increased pain when passively flexing and internally rotating the right hip. Several tests can be useful when evaluating a patient for appendicitis. McBurney point is where the right lower quadrant pain is best elicited. Rovsing sign is when pain is felt in the right lower quadrant when the left lower quadrant is palpated. Psoas sign is described in answer choice A, which increases pain due to stretching the iliopsoas muscle.

31. C: Sertraline. Tramadol should be used with caution when combined with selective serotonin reuptake inhibitors (SSRIs) because of the increased risk of seizures and serotonin syndrome. This also applies to serotonin-norepinephrine reuptake inhibitors (SNRIs), monoamine oxidase inhibitors (MAOIs), tricyclic antidepressants (TCAs), and triptans.

32. B: *Bordetella pertussis*. This disease is also known as whooping cough and can be prevented through immunization. It is very contagious and affects mostly children. Symptoms are generally nonspecific but the coughing itself has a characteristic "whoop" sound afterwards when the child inspires. Pertussis is treated with macrolide antibiotics. Hospitalization may be required as complications of the disease can be serious.

33. C: Peritonsillar abscess. Out of the listed conditions, this infection has the potential to be the most serious. It occurs when bacteria in the throat spread to the soft tissues. Patients may present with sore throat, "hot potato" voice, difficulty swallowing, fever, or earache. It is diagnosed with needle aspiration, and the abscess will need to be drained. Hospitalization may be required. A chalazion is a swelling of the eyelid caused by meibomian gland obstruction—it can improve spontaneously over time. Entropion is gradual inversion of the eyelid usually seen in elderly patients. Aphthous ulcers are also known as canker sores in the mouth.

34. D: 68-year-old woman with history of smoking. The major risk factors for development of abdominal aortic aneurysm (AAA) include male sex, smoking history, and age 65 or older. For men ages 65-75 with a smoking history, the benefits of screening outweigh the harms and the USPSTF gives this a "B" recommendation. For men ages 65-75 with no history of smoking, the USPSTF gives no recommendation

for or against screening. The USPSTF recommends against screening for AAA in women since there are few AAA-related deaths in this population.

35. C: Lyme disease. This infection is transmitted by ticks and is seen in those living in wooded areas. The rash is known as erythema migrans and is usually the first sign of infection. Rocky Mountain spotted fever is also a tick-borne illness that can occur in the United States. It presents with the same generalized symptoms, but the rash begins at the extremities and would include smaller macules. Erythema infectiosum is also known as fifth disease and is usually seen in children.

36. A: Congenital protrusion through the inguinal ring into inguinal canal. Answer choice B describes a direct inguinal hernia. Answer choice C describes a femoral hernia, and answer choice D describes an umbilical hernia.

37. C: 60 years old who had a normal Pap smear 5 years ago. The ACOG recommends that screening for cervical cancer should begin at age 21 regardless of when the patient became sexually active. For women ages 21-29, screening through cytology should occur every 3 years. Women ages 30-65 can be screened every 3 years through cytology or every 5 years with both cytology and HPV testing. Women older than 65 can stop screening if they have had 3 consecutive normal cytology tests and no abnormal results in the past 10 years.

38. D: Start levothyroxine. In patients with primary hypothyroidism, free $T_4$ is low and TSH is elevated. Levothyroxine is given to replace the thyroid hormone. The other answer options describe treatments for hyperthyroidism, in which the TSH would be low and free $T_4$ would usually be increased.

39. B: Attending more military events and talking about his experiences. The diagnostic criteria for PTSD include the following three symptom clusters that cause impairment for greater than a month following a traumatic event: re-experiencing, avoidance, and hyperarousal. Answer choice B does not fit with this because individuals with PTSD tend to avoid thoughts, feelings, places, and people that remind them of their trauma.

40. A: Furosemide. Diuretics increase urine volume. Furosemide is known as a loop diuretic and can cause hypokalemia. Triamterene and spironolactone are potassium-sparing diuretics, which means that they act by enhancing sodium excretion and retaining potassium in the distal tubule. Acetazolamide is a carbonic anhydrase inhibitor.

41. C: Osgood-Schlatter disease. This condition usually affects males between 10 and 15 years of age. It is thought to be caused by stress on the patellar tendon, which attaches to the tibial tuberosity. It is generally self-limited with conservative treatment. Slipped capital femoral epiphysis usually occurs in overweight adolescent boys, but affects the hip. Sever disease is also seen usually in young patients, but this affects the heels. Scheuermann disease affects the back.

42. A: Potassium hydroxide wet mount. Hyphae or budding yeast seen under a microscope can confirm candidiasis. This type of fungal infection can occur anywhere but is common in skinfolds, especially with hot weather and restrictive clothing. Biopsies are helpful when evaluating skin cancers. A Tzanck smear can help diagnose viral disease.

43. B: Advise use of compression stockings since she is on her feet all day. Varicose veins are dilated veins seen in the lower extremities. They can be painful and due to a number of causes, including venous insufficiency, genetics, prolonged standing, and pregnancy. Elevation of the legs can provide temporary

relief. Some patients opt for injection therapy or surgery, which can also be helpful from a cosmetic standpoint, although the problem can recur.

44. D: All of the above. Tourette disorder is a tic disorder that is usually first seen in childhood. It is a spectrum disorder and must be distinguished from transient tics or other conditions. Tics can be simple such as blinking or sniffing, or more complex such as vocalizations. For a diagnosis of Tourette disorder, multiple motor tics and at least one vocal tic must be present for a year. The tics are only temporarily suppressible. Treatment can include medications such as antipsychotics.

45. C: Antibiotic ointment for 5 days. This patient has a corneal abrasion, likely from improper use of contact lenses. Abrasions can present with a foreign body sensation. Antibiotic ointment is recommended to prevent infection. Irrigation is used when a foreign body is suspected or visualized. Eye patches and steroids are not used because they can worsen the condition.

46. A: Abductor pollicus longus and extensor pollicus brevis. The patient described has De Quervain syndrome, which is a tenosynovitis usually occurring due to overuse. These two muscles form the bulge on the lateral side of the wrist near the thumb, and the tendons form the lateral border of the anatomical snuffbox. A positive Finkelstein test elicits pain when adducting the wrist with the thumb tucked in the palm.

47. C: Blood. Infection is commonly transmitted with IV drug use, along with tattoos or body piercings. Transmission during sex and breastfeeding are relatively rare. Transmission of hepatitis B usually occurs through blood and sex. Hepatitis A spreads primarily by fecal-oral contact.

48. B: Counsel her that infertility is not diagnosed until after 1 year of unprotected intercourse. In the United States, women are not considered infertile until they have been trying to conceive for 12 months without contraception. It is generally recommended that women younger than age 30 wait until then to undergo further testing. Infertility can be due to factors in the female, male, or both.

49. D: Carbamazepine. Aplastic anemia occurs when there is a loss of blood cell precursors. The cause is unknown in most cases, but radiation, chemicals, and medications have been linked to the condition (benzene, certain antineoplastics, antibiotics, NSAIDS, and anticonvulsants). Carbamazepine is used as an anticonvulsant and mood stabilizer. Chloramphenicol is a rarely used antibiotic that has been associated with aplastic anemia.

50. C: Ménière disease. This condition is classically characterized by a triad of vertigo, fluctuating hearing loss, and tinnitus. Changes within the endolymph cause the patient's symptoms, although the root cause is not clear. Patients often have "attacks" consisting of the various symptoms. Medications and diet changes may be helpful in managing the condition. Some patients may require surgery due to debilitating episodes.

51. C: Catheter drainage. Pneumothorax can occur spontaneously, usually in thin, young males. Air in the pleural space can cause the lung volume to decrease and thus cause shortness of breath. It is diagnosed with x-ray. Small pneumothoraxes without symptoms can be observed with follow-up x-rays. A tension pneumothorax is when pressure is so great that the lung can collapse and shift the mediastinum—this is a medical emergency and needs to be treated immediately by inserting a catheter into the chest wall.

52. A: *E. coli*. This patient has cystitis, also known as a lower urinary tract infection. *E. coli* is responsible for roughly 90% of first infections in women. *Klebsiella, Enterobacter, Proteus, Pseudomonas*, and *Serratia* are also common. Culture is considered the gold standard for diagnosis but may not always be necessary.

53. C: Decreased hair growth. Cushing syndrome is due to adrenal hormone excess. Central obesity, "moon face," and thin skin with striae are due to changes in protein and fat metabolism. Patients with Cushing syndrome have excess hair growth due to changes in sex hormones, along with irregular periods and impotence.

54. D: Loss of skin melanocytes with unclear cause. This patient likely has vitiligo. It may be an autoimmune condition, although the true cause is unknown. There is a genetic component. Loss of skin melanocytes causes progressive areas of skin depigmentation. It commonly occurs on the face, digits, and flexor surfaces.

55. A: Beta-blockers. Hypertropic cardiomyopathy is a congenital disorder. Patients experience chest pain, shortness of breath, and syncope, and can have sudden death. It is diagnosed with echocardiography. Beta-blockers slow the heart rate, which prolongs the diastolic filling period, and ventricular diastolic function is improved. Nitrates and ACE inhibitors decrease chamber size and worsen the condition. Inotropes worsen outflow obstruction and may induce arrhythmias.

56. A: Steroids. Tetanus is also known as "lockjaw" and is caused by the neurotoxin from *Clostridium tetani*. Patients have tonic spasms of voluntary muscles. Disease is rare in the United States because of prevention through immunization. Immune globulin neutralizes the toxin, and metronidazole prevents further toxin release. Patients are also usually sedated to control muscles spasms. The wound should be debrided as well.

57. B: Pancreatitis. Endoscopic retrograde cholangiopancreatography (ERCP) is a procedure that uses x-ray to view the bile and pancreatic ducts. This procedure is often done because of a gallstone blockage. The scope is inserted through the mouth, and air is introduced so that the flexible tube can go into the lower structures. Mild pancreatitis occurs in 3% to 5% of people who undergo the procedure.

58. B: Acetylcholinesterase inhibitor. Patients with Alzheimer disease have a cerebral cholinergic deficit, and donepezil increases cholinergic transmission by inhibiting the enzyme that breaks down acetylcholine. It can improve cognition, behavior, and functioning with activities of daily living. Rivastigmine is an acetyl/butyrylcholinesterase inhibitor, galantamine is a cholinesterase and nicotinic receptor stimulation modulator, and memantine antagonizes glutamate.

59. A: Sinusitis. This condition is an inflammation or swelling of the sinuses. Patients present with rhinorrhea, anosmia, congestion, facial pain, headache, fever, and cough. Allergic rhinitis and nasal polyps may have similar symptoms, although sinus tenderness would not be present. Parotitis is an inflammation of the parotid gland.

60. D: Discharge with a low-dose antidepressant and make a close psychiatry follow-up appointment. Involuntary commitment to a hospital would be appropriate if a patient is considered to be a danger to self or others. With this patient, although he does have intermittent suicidal thoughts, he does not have current suicidal intent or plan. He declines voluntary hospitalization, so the best course of action is outpatient management. He could be discharged with a starting dose of an antidepressant as long as an outpatient mental health appointment can be ensured within the coming days.

61. C: Inferior vena cava. Greenfield inferior vena cava (IVC) filters, also known as venous filters, are implanted in patients with recurrent clots or in those who cannot take anticoagulants. The filter is cone-shaped and allows blood to flow around it, while trapping clots from the lower extremities before they reach the lungs.

62. D: "Tennis elbow." This is another name for lateral epicondylitis, which is caused by repetitive wrist extension. It involves the tendon for the extensor muscles of the wrist and hand. "Golfer's elbow" is also known as medial epicondylitis—pain would increase with wrist flexion. An ulnar collateral ligament tear would involve pain over the medial elbow. Olecranon bursitis would present with swelling.

63. A: < 100 mg/dL. In this patient, presence of DM and PVD are considered coronary heart disease equivalents, and he also has risk factors of being a cigarette smoker and older than 45 years. His LDL goal is < 100 mg/dL. For levels equal to or greater than 100 mg/dL, lifestyle changes should be initiated. For LDL levels equal to or greater than 130 mg/dL, drug therapy should be considered, although drug therapy is considered for some patients at a level of 100 mg/dL as well.

64. B: Pulmonary embolism. Risk factors include immobilization, recent surgery, malignancy, smoking, age, pregnancy, and diabetes. Most PEs involve the lower lobes. Chest x-ray may be normal or show atelectasis, pleural effusion, or infiltrate. A positive D-dimer is sensitive but not necessarily specific. The other answer choices listed could present similarly to this patient, but all of the factors combined, especially with recent surgery, make PE more likely. Pneumonia or CHF would likely have an abnormal chest x-ray. Acute MI would have elevated troponin.

65. A: The duration of symptoms will be reduced by 1 day. Oseltamivir is also known as *Tamiflu* and is a neuraminidase inhibitor, which competitively inhibits the surface viral protein. It is used for both prophylaxis and treatment. It can reduce the duration and severity of symptoms when initiated on the first day of illness. Patients should also undergo symptomatic therapy, such as using medications for fever and headache.

66. D: Testicular cancer. It usually occurs in white males between the ages of 18 and 30. It can progress rapidly, so diagnosis cannot be missed. A testicular mass can be felt that can be confirmed through ultrasound. Hydroceles are collections of fluid within the scrotum and usually painless. Spermatoceles are accumulations of sperm with no known etiology that are painless. Epididymitis usually presents with pain, edema, and erythema. In males younger than 35 years, epididymitis is usually concurrent with STDs.

67. C: Trichomoniasis. This condition is primarily sexually transmitted. Patients can present with vaginal discharge, pruritus, and dyspareunia. "Strawberry cervix" may be seen during pelvic exam, and parasites would be visible under the microscope. Metronidazole is an antibiotic that works well for protozoa. The partner must be treated too.

68. C: No treatment necessary as it will go away on its own. Pityriasis rosea usually affects patients between ages 10 and 35. This condition usually begins with a "herald" patch, and then oval papules will appear within 1 to 2 weeks. It may resemble ringworm. Lesions can be distributed in a "Christmas tree–like" pattern over the back. The condition will usually go away within 5 weeks without specific treatment.

69. D: All of the above. Hypertension can be primary (no known cause) or secondary (identifiable cause, usually renal disorders). It is defined as greater than or equal to systolic BP of 140 and/or diastolic BP of 90. Primary hypertension is believed to be due to multiple factors, including heredity and environment.

70. A: L2 to coccyx. The cauda equina ("horsetail") consists of the spinal nerves in the area below the conus medullaris (at level L1) of the spinal cord. An injury at L1 or above will damage the spinal cord itself. Cauda equina damage can include motor loss, diminished sensation in the perineal region, and bowel/bladder impairment. It may be caused by trauma, spinal stenosis, ruptured disk, or tumor. It requires urgent surgical treatment.

71. B: $H_2$ receptor antagonist. Ranitidine is used in the treatment of gastroesophageal reflux disease (GERD) and peptic ulcer disease. It blocks histamine on parietal cells in the stomach and thus decreases acid production. In the United States, it is now available over the counter. Antihistamines used for allergy symptoms are $H_1$ receptor antagonists.

72. A: Kerley B lines. These markings on chest x-ray signify pulmonary edema. They appear as short parallel lines at the edges of the lungs or costophrenic angles, and they indicate thickening of the septa. With CHF, you would expect the heart to be enlarged. Ground glass appearance is usually seen with interstitial disease. Silhouette sign is when the border of a structure cannot be viewed, like with atelectasis when the lung lobe obscures the heart.

73. C: Epiglottitis. This is a bacterial infection of the epiglottis and surrounding structures that requires emergent care because of possibility of asphyxia. It may occur in children or adults. Drooling is common, and the patient may be in a "tripod position," leaning forward in order to breathe. Differential diagnosis could include croup, airway foreign body, and peritonsillar abscess. A "beefy red" epiglottis seen on laryngoscopy is diagnostic of epiglottitis.

74. B: Fallopian tube. An ectopic pregnancy is when implantation occurs anywhere outside the endometrium. Patients may present with pain and bleeding during early pregnancy. Risk increases with advanced maternal age, PID, and smoking. The second most common site is the uterine interstitium.

75. D: MRI. Optic neuritis is an inflammation of the optic nerve that can present with sudden vision loss and pain. The most common cause is multiple sclerosis, which can show up on an MRI as demyelination. MRI is the most sensitive test for multiple sclerosis (MS). Other less common causes of optic neuritis include infection and autoimmune disorders, such as lupus.

76. C: Low-dose inhaled corticosteroid daily. This patient falls into the "mild persistent" class of asthma sufferers (daytime symptoms more than 2 times per week, nighttime symptoms more than 2 times per month, exacerbations that sometimes limit activity). Treatment of asthma is a stepwise approach. For patients with mild intermittent asthma, no daily drugs are required, and rescue beta-agonists can be used as needed. For patients older than 5 years with mild persistent asthma, low-dose inhaled corticosteroids are recommended along with rescue beta-agonists.

77. D: Intubation and general anesthesia. Status epilepticus is when the brain is in a continuous state of seizure for at least 5 minutes. It requires drugs to terminate the seizure and monitoring of respiratory status. If patients continue to seize after administration of lorazepam and phenytoin, they are considered to have refractory status epilepticus, and a third anticonvulsant is usually given. Intubation is necessary if the airway is compromised or if the seizure has not terminated at this point.

78. B: Proportions are not normal. Hypopituitarism in children can result in short stature, also known as dwarfism. A pituitary tumor is usually the cause, but it also may be idiopathic. Growth hormone is decreased. Proportions are normal, unlike short-limbed dwarfism that is seen due to osteochondrodysplasias.

79. A: HbA$_{1c}$. Quetiapine is in the antipsychotic class of medications, which can be used to treat mood disorders and psychotic disorders. Other drugs in this class include risperidone, aripiprazole, ziprasidone, and olanzapine. Blood glucose, blood pressure, cholesterol, and weight need to be monitored regularly when patients on are these medications because of the potential metabolic side effects. Patients should also be monitored for abnormal movements, such as tardive dyskinesia.

80. B: ST segment abnormality. An acute myocardial infarction is when coronary arteries become obstructed, resulting in cardiac ischemia. The patient's symptoms can include chest pain, shortness of breath, and diaphoresis. An ECG will make the diagnosis, along with markers such as troponin and myocardial-bound creatine phosphokinase (CPK-MB).

81. B: NSAIDs. Osteoarthritis is also known as degenerative joint disease. Patients are more likely to experience osteoarthritis as they get older. It can occur in the hands, hips, knees, and feet. Osteoarthritis begins with tissue damage, inflammation, or defects in cartilage metabolism. NSAIDs or acetaminophen can help relieve pain. Muscle relaxants and narcotics tend to cause more side effects, especially in elderly patients.

82. A: Rubbery prostate with digital rectal exam. Benign prostatic hyperplasia can cause urinary frequency, urgency, nocturia, hesitancy, and dribbling. BPH etiology is unknown, but may be related to changes in hormones due to aging. BPH patients would have a "rubbery" prostate, whereas patients with prostate cancer may have a hard, nodular prostate. Fever and elevated white blood cell count would be more common with an infection like prostatitis.

83. D: Molluscum contagiosum. This condition is caused by a virus and can be spread by contact. Most lesions will go away on their own. Milia are keratin-filled cysts that usually occur around the nose and eyes. Warts are also caused by a virus but are rougher in appearance and may have an irregular shape. Folliculitis is an inflammation of the hair follicles and may look more like pustules.

84. B: Delayed childbearing. Endometriosis is when tissue is implanted outside the uterine cavity, causing pain and infertility. It is diagnosed with biopsy. Incidence is increased with delayed childbearing, family history of endometriosis, shortened menstrual cycles, and abnormally long periods. Protective factors seem to be multiple pregnancies and use of contraceptives.

85. C: Pericardiocentesis. Pericarditis is an inflammation of the sac around the heart that can be caused by MI, trauma, or infection, or the cause may be unknown. When pericarditis involves a large effusion and impairs cardiac filling, it is known as cardiac tamponade and can lead to shock and death. It is treated immediately with pericardiocentesis in order to remove fluid from around the heart.

86. D: 24-28 weeks. Gestational diabetes increases morbidity and mortality of both mother and fetus, so all pregnant women are screened with an oral glucose tolerance test. Women with risk factors such as prior gestational diabetes, unexplained fetal losses, family history of diabetes, or BMI more than 30 may be screened in the first trimester.

87. A: Amitriptyline. This medication is a tricyclic antidepressant, which can have significant anticholinergic side effects such as constipation, weight gain, dizziness, urinary retention, and blurred vision. Amitriptyline may worsen glaucoma and should be used with caution in elderly patients.

88. B: Arthrocentesis. Gout occurs when monosodium urate crystals deposit into tissue. Patients usually present with a painful, warm, red metatarsophalangeal joint. Uric acid levels may be elevated, but not all people with elevated uric acid levels develop gout. An x-ray may be more useful when identifying tophi in chronic gout. ESR is not specific for gout. Definitive diagnosis is done by arthrocentesis, which will show monosodium urate crystals in the synovial fluid.

89. D: Growth regulators cause hepatocellular hypoplasia. Cirrhosis occurs because of chronic liver disease. Normal hepatic structure progresses to fibrosis and disorganization of tissue. Cytokines and

growth regulators actually induce hepatocellular hyperplasia in response to injury. This produces regenerating nodules and angiogenesis.

90. C: Palliative care should be discussed. Cystic fibrosis is an inherited disease that primarily affects the respiratory and GI systems. Treatment is supportive, including infection prevention, chest physical therapy, diet changes, and management of associated conditions. Transplantation often becomes necessary, although the patient should be given options and information regarding quality of life. The median survival age is in the late 30s.

91. C: Tell them to avoid smoking as this is the biggest risk factor. Oral squamous cell carcinoma may occur on the floor of the mouth, tongue, lip, or palate. Smoking and alcohol use are the biggest risk factors for development of this condition. It can be detected early by screening, with biopsies of suspicious areas. It is treated with surgery and/or radiation.

92. D: Guillain-Barré syndrome. This condition is an inflammatory neuropathy that presents as muscle weakness and sensory loss. The cause it thought to be autoimmune, with an infection sometimes being the trigger. Most patients improve within several months. A stroke would usually cause weakness just on one side of the body. Myasthenia gravis also presents with weakness, although the symptoms worsen with exertion. Amyotrophic lateral sclerosis, also known as Lou Gehrig disease, presents with more asymmetric weakness.

93. B: Mupirocin ointment. Based on the information given, this patient likely has impetigo—a bacterial skin infection usually caused by staphylococci or streptococci. It commonly begins as a sore near the nose or mouth, with pus leading to formation of a honey-colored crust. It may be itchy and is highly contagious. Mupirocin is an antibiotic.

94. C: Reduction in brain volume. Schizophrenia is a complex mental disorder characterized by psychosis, disorganization, flattened affect, and cognitive deficits. There is a genetic component, although the full cause is unknown. Some studies have shown that patients with schizophrenia have a reduction in brain volume along with enlarged lateral and third ventricles.

95. A: Kidney. Wilms tumor, also known as nephroblastoma, is an embryonal cancer of the kidney. It usually presents in children younger than 5 years. Patients may have a painless abdominal mass with hematuria, fever, nausea, and vomiting. It is diagnosed with CT and biopsy. Treatment includes surgery, chemotherapy, and radiation.

96. D: Bone pain. Multiple myeloma is a malignancy in which abnormal plasma cells accumulate in bone marrow, leading to bone pain, renal insufficiency, and anemia. Lytic bone lesions may be seen on x-ray. The breakdown of bone leads to hypercalcemia. Patients are more susceptible to infections due to decreased production of immunoglobulin. It is treated with chemotherapy and stem cell transplantation.

97. A: Azithromycin. This patient likely has chlamydia, which is a common sexually transmitted infection. Infected men will present with urethritis and a clear or cloudy discharge. Sexual partners should be treated as well. Azithromycin is a macrolide antibiotic. Untreated chlamydia can lead to more serious health problems.

98. C: When hemorrhoids fail to respond to more conservative measures. Hemorrhoids are dilated veins in the rectum that can be asymptomatic or cause pain and bleeding. Hemorrhoids can be internal or external, sometimes protruding from the anus. They can thrombose, resulting in painful swelling. Patients should use stool softeners, take warm baths, apply anesthetic ointments, and take OTC medications for

pain. Incision/evacuation, injection sclerotherapy, and ligation are also treatment options. Hemorrhoidectomy is done for patients who do not respond to these other therapies.

99. B: Diverticulitis. Patients with low-fiber diets may have diverticulosis, which consists of outpouchings of the colon. When these become inflamed or perforate, patients develop diverticulitis, which usually presents with pain in the left lower quadrant and fever. Patients may develop abscesses or bowel obstructions. Patients with severe symptoms are hospitalized and given IV fluids and antibiotics. Surgery may be necessary in patients with perforation.

100. B: Glargine. Diabetes can be treated by administration of exogenous insulin, due to the patient no longer producing insulin internally or the patient being insulin resistant. Glargine has a duration of action of roughly 18-26 hours. Aspart and lispro are fast-acting insulins, and NPH is an intermediate-acting insulin.

101. A: Acute bacterial endocarditis. This patient likely has an infection of the endocardium, which is the inner layer of the heart. IV drug use, recent dental procedures, and prior heart valve issues increase the risk of developing endocarditis. Usually caused by streptococci or staphylococci, "vegetations" form on the heart valves. Patients present with fever, heart murmur, and evidence of emboli from the infected material on the valve. It is diagnosed by blood culture and echocardiography. It is treated with IV antibiotics and may require surgery.

102. B: Decreased gonadotropin secretion. This patient has primary amenorrhea, which is the absence of menarche by age 16. Gonadotropins are hormones such as LH and follicle-stimulating hormone (FSH) that are secreted by the pituitary gland and act on the ovaries. Decreased gonadotropin secretion results in estrogen deficiency—this is the most common reason for amenorrhea. Increased testosterone may also lead to amenorrhea, as may be seen with polycystic ovary syndrome.

103. D: None of the above. Based on the information provided, this patient has a pterygium, which is a benign growth of the conjunctiva. It is diagnosed by physical examination and does not require any specific tests. The pterygium may eventually spread across the cornea and distort vision. It can be removed to improve vision or for cosmetic purposes.

104. C: Sildenafil. This medication is a phosphodiesterase type 5 (PDE5) inhibitor that is used to treat erectile dysfunction, but it is contradicted when patients are already taking nitrates. Isosorbide dinitrate and sildenafil are both vasodilators and can cause hypotension when used in conjunction.

105. A: 65. The most common bacterial cause of pneumonia in the United States is *Streptococcus pneumoniae*, also known as pneumococcus. Symptoms include fever, cough, and shortness of breath. Elderly patients are at greater risk for pneumococcal disease. The pneumococcal vaccine (PCV13) is routinely given to infants in a series of four doses. The pneumococcal vaccine (PPSV) is recommended for all adults 65 years and older if they received their first dose before age 65 and if it has been 5 or more years since their first dose. Older children and adults younger than 65 are also vaccinated if they have certain medical conditions.

106. B: Primidone. This medication is an anticonvulsant. This patient has essential tremor, which is benign and usually associated with older age. It may be hereditary. It can also be treated with beta-blockers, such as propranolol. A tremor associated with Parkinson disease would be present at rest and decrease with activity.

107. D: Ganglion cyst. These usually occur on the dorsal aspect of the hand or wrist. They are more common in women between 20 and 50 years of age. The cause is unknown. The cysts are usually attached to tendon sheaths and joint capsules. They may be removed surgically. Tenosynovitis would not present with a well-circumscribed mass. With gout, the joint would be red and painful.

108. B: Frequent sun exposure. Actinic keratosis is a condition usually seen in fair-skinned people with frequent sun exposure. It is considered to be premalignant, meaning that the areas could progress to squamous cell carcinoma. Patients will have scaly/crusty, pink areas of skin usually on sun-exposed areas such as the face. It can be treated with medications, laser resurfacing, or cryotherapy.

109. D: A 26-year-old woman who is breastfeeding. Mastitis is an inflammation of the breast, usually with infection by staphylococci, streptococci, or *E. coli*. It is a common maternal complication of breastfeeding due to engorgement and blockage. Patients present with fever and a red, swollen, painful area of the breast. Treatment includes antibiotics and continued breastfeeding in order to empty the breast.

110. B: Chest CT. There are many causes for solitary pulmonary nodules, including cysts, arteriovenous malformations, tuberculosis, hematomas, and neoplasms. Lesions may be benign or malignant. Risks factors for lung cancer include age, smoking, asbestos exposure, and family history. Certain lesion characteristics, such as an irregular border, may be indicative of a malignancy. It is best to evaluate risk factors for each patient and do a thorough history/physical. It is helpful to compare with old imaging if available to determine if the lesion has grown. A chest CT is a reasonable next step for this patient in order to better characterize the lesion. If there is concern for malignancy, then excision or biopsy would be done.

111. B: Decreasing physical activity. Osteoporosis is a condition in which bone density is decreased, which can lead to fractures. It is more common in women and elderly patients. White and Asian patients are at higher risk, along with those who have a family history of osteoporosis. Exercise is actually recommended because the weight-bearing and stress are necessary for bone growth. Goals with treatment are to preserve bone mass, prevent fractures, and decrease pain. Bisphosphonates work by inhibiting bone resorption.

112. A: Lorazepam. Alcohol withdrawal can be potentially fatal. Symptoms of withdrawal are usually 12-48 hours after last drink. Patients may have stomach upset, tremor, weakness, and sweating. Delirium tremens (DTs) can occur within 48-72 hours and include increasing anxiety, confusion, hallucinations, and autonomic lability. Benzodiazepines are used to treat alcohol withdrawal because they are CNS depressants, like alcohol. They should not be continued after the detoxification period because of their risk of dependence as well.

113. D: Indomethacin. Patent ductus arteriosus (PDA) is when the aorta and pulmonary artery are still connected after birth. Infants may be poor feeders and have tachycardia and tachypnea. A murmur can be heard. For premature infants, indomethacin may close the PDA since prostaglandin E2 is responsible for keeping the ductus patent. Indomethacin is a prostaglandin synthesis inhibitor/NSAID. If indomethacin is ineffective, surgery can be done.

114. C: High. Presbyacusis is bilateral, symmetric, sensorineural hearing loss due to normal aging. It usually affects the highest frequencies (18-20 kHz) and can impair speech comprehension. High-frequency hearing loss is also caused by noise damage. The results of a hearing test are displayed in an audiogram, which shows the level that sounds are detected at each frequency.

115. B: There are numerous potential etiologies. Dilated cardiomyopathy leads to heart failure due to enlargement of the ventricles. Systolic function is mainly affected. There are many potential causes of this condition, including coronary artery disease (CAD) and viruses. Patients have shortness of breath, fatigue, and peripheral edema. Restrictive cardiomyopathy means that the ventricular walls are noncompliant and diastolic filling is limited. Causes of restrictive cardiomyopathy include amyloidosis, sarcoidosis, and hemochromatosis. Patients have shortness of breath on exertion and fatigue.

116. D: Nephrolithiasis. Patients with kidney stones may have sudden onset of unilateral flank pain, hematuria, abdominal pain, nausea, urgency, frequency, or dysuria. Pyelonephritis is an infection of the kidney. Patients may also have dysuria, flank pain, and nausea, but they would also have fever and an elevated white blood cell count. Patient with BPH have urinary frequency and urgency, but would not typically have back pain or hematuria. Prostatitis would likely present with urinary frequency and urgency, fever, and sometimes testicular or perineal pain.

117. C: Acute bronchitis. Coughs and bronchitis are usually caused by viruses and do not require antibiotics for treatment. The upper airway is inflamed and fever may not be present, unlike pneumonia in which the lungs are involved and patients have fever. Allergic rhinitis presents with congestion, sore throat, cough, and itchy/watery eyes. "Cobblestoning" may be seen in the pharynx due to postnasal drip, and eyes may be affected. Sinus infections are usually accompanied by facial pain and headache.

118. A: Cholecystitis. Inflammation of the gallbladder presents with pain in the upper right quadrant. A positive Murphy sign is when this pain can be elicited with patient inspiration when the examiner's hand palpates under the ribs on the right side.

119. A: Prompt delivery. Abruptio placentae is when the placenta prematurely separates from the uterus during late pregnancy. Patients can present with bleeding and pain. Severity depends on the degree of separation, but it can lead to fetal distress and maternal shock. It is diagnosed clinically or with ultrasound. Mild symptoms may be treated with bed rest, but prompt delivery is more appropriate when the life of mother or fetus is threatened.

120. B: Antibiotics. Stevens-Johnson syndrome is a potentially life-threatening hypersensitivity reaction in which patients present with ulcers, widespread macules, and blistering. It can be caused by drugs (sulfa drugs, antiepileptics, antibiotics), infections, or vaccinations. Treatment is supportive.

121. D: Contacting Adult Protective Services. All of these answer choices are appropriate steps to take in management of this patient; however, contacting APS is obligatory for health care professionals who suspect that a patient is being abused or neglected. This patient is at risk because of dementia, and there are signs of abuse/neglect such as bruising and poor hygiene.

122. C: Mebendazole. This medication is an antihelminthic. This patient has pinworms, which is an intestinal parasitic infection common in children. It is transmitted from human to human by contamination and ingestion. It presents as anal itching, usually worse at night because this is when the female pinworm migrates to lay eggs around the anus. Sometimes the worms are visible upon inspection.

123. D: Deficiency of pulmonary surfactant. Hyaline membrane disease is also known as neonatal respiratory distress syndrome. The risk for this condition depends on how premature the infant is. Surfactant diminishes the surface tension of lung alveoli, increasing pulmonary compliance and preventing lung collapse. Infants with deficiency of surfactant become hypoxemic and have more difficulty breathing.

124. B: Patients present with the same symptoms. For both STEMI and NSTEMI, patients can present with the same symptoms of angina, shortness of breath, fatigue, diaphoresis, and nausea. NSTEMI has subendocardial ischemia, where STEMI has transmural ischemia that extends through the whole thickness of the heart muscle. For NSTEMI, emergency percutaneous coronary intervention (PCI) is not necessarily indicated unless patient is high risk—with hemodynamic instability or elevated cardiac markers.

125. A: Avoid alcohol. Gout is due to monosodium urate crystals precipitating into tissue. Increased use of alcohol and red meats tend to make the condition worse. NSAIDs can actually prevent and provide relief for gout attacks. Physical activity does not necessarily make gout worse, and it has shown to be helpful.

126. D: Aortic dissection. Tears in the layers of the aorta cause intense pain. The dissection may extend along the aorta and into other arteries. The DeBakey classification system indicates the location and extent of the dissection. Hypertension is the main risk factor for development of this condition.

127. B: *C. difficile. Clostridium difficile* is a spore-forming gram-positive bacillus. It is the leading cause of nosocomial infectious diarrhea. The biggest risk factor for development is antibiotic use, especially fluoroquinolones and clindamycin. The antibiotics disturb the colonic flora. Individuals are also at greater risk if they are older than 65, have medical comorbidities, have irritable bowel disease, or are immunocompromised. Symptoms include fever, abdominal cramping, and watery diarrhea with mucus. Blood is not usually present.

128. D: Topical mydriatic agents. Strabismus is when the eyes are misaligned. Patient will have gaze deviation. It may be diagnosed clinically in children at routine visits. The corneal light reflex test can be used for detection. Topical miotic agents are used instead in the management of this condition because they cause constriction of the pupil and help with accommodation.

129. B: Rosacea. This is a chronic inflammatory disorder that usually affects patients between 30 and 50 years of age. Treatment involves avoidance of triggers (such as sun, stress, alcohol, wind, cosmetics) and antibiotics. Psoriasis is also an inflammatory disease, but the lesions are usually better circumscribed and have silvery scales. Erysipelas is superficial cellulitis that could present as distinct, shiny plaque lesions on the face. It is usually accompanied by fever. Melasma consists of dark, irregular macules usually occurring in pregnant women.

130. C: A 24-year-old woman with upper respiratory tract infection and fever. Influenza is a common viral infection seen between the months of October and May. Cases peak around January and February. The vaccine is not approved for infants younger than 6 months, but is otherwise universally recommended. However, if patients are moderately to severely ill with fever, they should wait to be vaccinated until after their symptoms diminish. The vaccine is especially recommended for those at greater risk of flu complications, such as those younger than 5 years, greater than 50 years, living in a nursing home, those who are pregnant, or have chronic medical conditions.

131. A: Low calcium. Hypoparathyroidism can be caused by surgical removal or incidental destruction of the parathyroid glands. Inadequate parathyroid hormone results in hypocalcemia. Patients can have vague or neuromuscular symptoms. Chronic hypocalcemia can lead to mental status changes, cataracts, dry skin, and brittle hair/nails.

132. A: GI bleed. Nonsteroidal anti-inflammatory drugs can be used for acute or chronic pain. They are not narcotics. NSAIDs irritate the gastric mucosa and reduce the level of protective prostaglandins. Patients may experiences nausea, vomiting, dyspepsia, or bleeding.

133. B: Increasing age. Gender is actually the biggest risk factor, followed by increasing age. For women in their 20s, approximately 1 in 2000 will develop breast cancer, compared with 1 in 25 for women 70 years and older. Other risk factors include family history or personal history of breast cancer, estrogen exposure, earlier menarche, later menopause, fewer pregnancies, and no history of breastfeeding.

134. C: G6PD deficiency. This is an X-linked hereditary disease more common in black patients, characterized by abnormally low levels of glucose-6-phosphate dehydrogenase, which is a metabolic enzyme. Deficiency leads to reduced energy available to maintain RBC membranes. Hemolysis can occur after acute illness or use of certain medications. Heinz bodies are inclusions within RBCs composed of denatured hemoglobin. When macrophages remove the Heinz bodies, characteristic "bite cells" are left.

135. A: Right atrium, right ventricle, left atrium, left ventricle. Blood comes into the right atrium by way of the superior vena cava and inferior vena cave. It goes through the tricuspid valve into the right ventricle, where it is then pumped to the lungs to become oxygenated. Blood returns into the left atrium and flows through the mitral valve into the left ventricle. It is then pumped throughout the body.

136. C: Patent foramen ovale. This patient likely has a type of atrial septal defect known as a patent foramen ovale. During fetal development, the foramen ovale is open so that blood flows between the atria and bypasses the nonfunctional lungs. It is congenital, although some patients may not present with symptoms until later in life. Most small atrial septal defects (ASDs) are asymptomatic or will close within the first few years of life. With larger defects, a left-to-right shunt is present, which produces dyspnea, fatigue, and exercise intolerance.

137. D: Administer 100% oxygen. This patient is suffering from a cluster headache, which primarily affects men between 20 and 40 years of age. The exact cause is unknown. The excruciating headaches occur suddenly with autonomic symptoms on the same side. It is treated acutely with oxygen, and there are medications that patients can take to prevent the attacks.

138. A: It can be caused by stress or anxiety. Erectile dysfunction is the inability to attain or sustain an erection. The causes for ED include vascular, neurologic, hormonal, and psychological disorders. In the United States, 10-20 million men are affected. Prevalence increases with age. The treatment is with phosphodiesterase type 5 inhibitors, which prevent the degradation of cyclic GMP (cGMP). Increased cGMP results in vasodilation and increased blood flow.

139. D: Rh-negative mother who gave birth to an Rh-positive baby. The injection of Rh immune globulin is given to Rh-negative women who deliver an Rh-positive baby. The injection prevents the mother's immune system from forming antibodies against Rh-positive blood cells, which entered the bloodstream due to fetal circulation. The injection prevents hemolytic disease of the newborn, which can occur in subsequent pregnancies also.

140. B: Aortic stenosis. This patient presents with the classic triad of symptoms. Aortic stenosis is when the valve is narrowed between the left ventricle and the aorta, so a murmur is heard whenever blood is flowing out to the body. Untreated, this condition can lead to heart failure and arrhythmias. Treatment is with valve replacement.

141. D: Positive HIV. Kaposi sarcoma is a type of tumor that often occurs in AIDS patients, originating from infection with herpes virus. Immunosuppression increases the likelihood that patients will develop this tumor. Patients usually have multiple cutaneous lesions, and sometimes this is their first manifestation of AIDS.

142. B: Treat supportively. This patient likely has mononucleosis, which is caused by the Epstein-Barr virus. Antibiotics only work for bacterial infections. In this case, treatment is supportive and the condition is usually self-limited. Patients may have symptoms for weeks or months, including fatigue, fever, and lymphadenopathy. It is usually spread by human contact via asymptomatic viral shedding. There is the potential for complications with this condition, including splenic rupture.

143. D: Long-acting beta-agonist. Emphysema and chronic bronchitis are types of chronic obstructive pulmonary disease (COPD), usually related to cigarette smoking. With emphysema, patient's lungs have lost elastic recoil and are hyperinflated. Beta-agonists relax bronchial smooth muscle.

144. B: Typically begin above the renal arteries. AAAs usually are below the renal arteries. Risk factors for development of an AAA include male sex, smoking, and older age. Most are asymptomatic but carry the risk of eventually rupturing.

145. D: Pelvic inflammatory disease. This condition may be due to sexually transmitted diseases. Microorganisms spread into the upper female genital tract, which can cause pain, discharge, and fever. Diagnosis is suspected clinically in women of reproductive age with risk factors such as multiple sex partners. Patients are treated with antibiotics to cover gonorrhea and chlamydia. Patients may require hospitalization.

146. D: Fluorescein staining. Corneal abrasions can be caused by trauma, improper contact lens wear, and foreign bodies. Patients will experience pain, tearing, and redness. After using a topical anesthetic, fluorescein stain and a cobalt blue light can be used to illuminate abrasions. Corneal abrasions are treated with antibiotics. A CT may be necessary if an intraocular foreign body is suspected.

147. B: Exposure therapy. This patient has a specific phobia of dogs, which consists of an unreasonable and persistent fear that leads to anxiety and avoidance. With the help of a trained clinician, exposure therapy involves having patients face progressively stronger stimuli in a hierarchy, in order to overcome their anxiety. Cognitive processing therapy is usually used in treatment of PTSD, and dialectical behavior therapy is used to treat borderline personality disorder. Psychodynamic therapy is similar to psychoanalysis.

148. A: Upper abdomen, radiating to the back. Pancreatitis is usually due to biliary tract disease or excessive alcohol use. Pain may be reduced with leaning forward and worsened by coughing. Patients usually also have nausea and vomiting. It is diagnosed with amylase and lipase levels. Treatment is supportive.

149. C: Reactive arthritis. Formerly known as Reiter syndrome, this is an autoimmune condition that occurs after an initial infection. The initial infection may be sexually transmitted or gastrointestinal. The classic triad of symptoms includes arthritis, conjunctivitis, and urethritis. It usually affects men 20-40 years of age. There may be a genetic predisposition.

150. B: Congestive heart failure. Brain natriuretic peptide (BNP) is secreted by the heart ventricles in response to excessive stretching. The release of this polypeptide is intended to decrease systemic vascular resistance, increase urine production, and lower blood pressure. For patients with congestive

- 167 -

heart failure, BNP is usually over 100. The left and/or right ventricular dysfunction of heart failure can cause shortness of breath and peripheral edema. BNP may also be elevated in patients with renal dysfunction.

151. B: Small cell lung carcinoma. The other answer choices are types of non–small cell lung carcinoma (NSCLC), which comprise the majority of lung cancers. Small cell lung carcinomas (SCLCs) account for about 15% of lung cancers. In SCLCs, the cells contain neurosecretory granules and may result in paraneoplastic syndromes. SCLC usually begins near the center of the chest. This cancer grows quickly, and patients may present with metastatic disease. It is almost always caused by smoking. Patients present with hemoptysis, shortness of breath, and weight loss. It can be complicated with superior vena cava syndrome due to compression or invasion. Treatment is with chemotherapy and radiation, although prognosis is generally poor.

152. D: Median. This patient has carpal tunnel syndrome (CTS), which is caused by compression of the median nerve. Patients present with paresthesia and pain. It can be unilateral or bilateral. Phalen test is when you ask a patient to put the backs of their hands together, flexing the wrists. This maneuver increases the pressure in the carpal tunnel and symptoms should be elicited if the patient has CTS. It can be treated with surgery.

153. D: Chronic otitis media. A cholesteatoma is an epithelial cell growth in the middle ear, which can lead to hearing loss and further infection. Patients will have white debris in the middle ear and drainage. Surgery may be necessary because of potential serious complications and recurrence. It can affect patients of any age. Cholesteatomas can also be congenital.

154. C: 18-25. Epiphyseal plates are also known as growth plates and are present at the end of long bones. They are growing zones of cartilage, and the process of bone growth is known as ossification. The epiphyseal plates are replaced by epiphyseal lines when growth is complete—cartilage is replaced by bone, fusing the epiphyses and diaphysis.

155. B: 5 mm. Patients with kidney stones present with flank pain and hematuria. Stones have varying compositions, sizes, and locations. They are diagnosed by noncontrast CT, which can show location and severity of obstruction. For stones less than 5 mm in size, treatment is focused on pain management. Smaller stones usually pass with time. Larger stones have to be surgically removed.

156. A: Acute peripheral arterial occlusion. Whenever an artery gets blocked, patients present with the "Ps"—pain, pallor, pulselessness, paresthesia, and polar (cold). This patient likely has underlying peripheral arterial disease (PAD), which is due to atherosclerosis, and symptoms depend on the degree of obstruction. Risk factors include hypertension, hyperlipidemia, diabetes, and cigarette smoking. Mild PAD will cause intermittent claudication.

157. B: It occurs most often among Jewish patients. Phenylketonuria (PKU) is a genetic condition characterized by elevated phenylalanine due to an enzyme deficiency. It is most common in white populations. The mousy odor is due to a breakdown product of phenylalanine. It may present with seizures, gait disturbance, or hyperactivity. Untreated PKU can lead to intellectual disability. Treatment involves restricting phenylalanine in diet.

158. A: Gentamicin. This is in the aminoglycoside class of antibiotics that has been known to cause ototoxicity in some patients, which can manifest as hearing loss or disequilibrium. Other aminoglycoside antibiotics include streptomycin and tobramycin. Some macrolide antibiotics have also been linked with

ototoxicity. Amoxicillin is a penicillin antibiotic, levofloxacin is a quinolone, and cefprozil is a cephalosporin.

159. B: Colchicine. This medication is an anti-inflammatory and can be used for both prophylaxis and treatment of acute gout attacks. Allopurinol is a xanthine oxidase inhibitor. Xanthine oxidase is responsible for the production of uric acid, so allopurinol helps to lower uric levels and prevent future gout attacks. Allopurinol is not helpful in alleviating acute gout attacks. Methotrexate is used to treat rheumatoid arthritis, and azathioprine is an immunosuppressant.

160. D: Heart apex. Mitral regurgitation occurs when blood flows back into the left atrium during systole when the left ventricle contracts. Patients have shortness of breath, fatigue, and palpitations. The murmur is holosystolic, and it may be high or low pitched depending on the severity. The murmur may increase with handgrip or squatting.

161. C: Yes, start Metformin. A patient is now considered to have diabetes if their hemoglobin $A_{1c}$ is 6.5% or higher. Metformin is in the biguanide class of medications and is considered first-line treatment in those diagnosed with diabetes. It reduces complications and mortality. The main side effect can be gastrointestinal upset. Insulin or other medications may become necessary for some patients who are not able to maintain glucose control on metformin alone.

162. D: Seborrheic dermatitis. The other answer choices are all plausible diagnoses because they can all present with similar symptoms. Urticaria, also known as hives, has many causes. The wheals are red and itchy. Atopic dermatitis also presents with itchiness and erythema. It is an immune-mediated condition. Contact dermatitis is also a possible diagnosis. It is an acute inflammation that can be caused by various irritants, including poison ivy. Seborrheic dermatitis is less plausible as a diagnosis because this occurs where sebaceous glands are present, such as on the face and scalp. It causes dandruff and greasy scaling.

163. C: Adolescents and adults at increased risk and pregnant women. The USPSTF has an "A (strong) recommendation" to screen for HIV in adolescents and adults at increased risk for infection. Risk factors include men who have had sex with men after 1975, men and women with multiple partners, IV drug use, exchanging sex for money, infected partners, and blood transfusion between 1978 and 1985. A person is also considered to be high risk if they receive health care in a high-risk clinical setting, such as a correctional facility or homeless shelter. The USPSTF makes no recommendation for or against screening in adolescents and adults who are not at increased risk. The USPSTF also has an "A (strong) recommendation" for screening all pregnant women.

164. A: Elevated angiotensin-converting enzyme. Sarcoidosis is a condition with an unknown cause that can affect many organ systems. It is characterized by the presence of granulomas in tissue, most often affecting the lungs. The granulomas produce ACE. Elevated ACE is suggestive of diagnosis but can also be nonspecific. Calcium may be elevated because of production of vitamin D analogs. Leukopenia can occur due to a decreased number of circulating lymphocytes. Renal and hepatic involvement can lead to abnormal test results.

165. D: All of the above. Atrial fibrillation is an irregularly irregular heartbeat characterized by weakness, shortness of breath, and palpitations. It is one of the most common arrhythmias. Other causes include congenital heart disorders, COPD, and pericarditis. Stroke can be a complication, so part of treatment involves blood thinners for prevention.

166. B: Pressured speech, grandiose, flight of ideas. The mental status examination is used in the field of psychiatry to describe the characteristics of patients through observation and questioning. It includes

- 169 -

documentation of appearance, attitude, motor activity, speech, affect, mood, thought process, perception, insight, and judgment. Patients with bipolar disorder in a manic state likely have high energy, irritability, delusions of grandeur, and decreased need for sleep. Answer choice A is more descriptive of a patient with a psychotic disorder. Answer choice C describes a depressed patient, and answer choice D describes an anxious patient.

167. C: Mirtazapine. This medication works for both depression and anxiety symptoms and is best taken at night because sedation is a common side effect. Mirtazapine is also known to increase appetite. Bupropion is a norepinephrine-dopamine reuptake inhibitor, and venlafaxine is a serotonin-norepinephrine reuptake inhibitor. Both of these medications can also help depression/anxiety, but are best taken in the morning because they can cause activation or insomnia. Citalopram is another SSRI.

168. D: Pheochromocytoma. This is a cause of secondary hypertension. It is a tumor of the adrenal glands that secretes catecholamines and leads to persistent hypertension. It usually occurs in patients between 20 and 40 years of age. There is a hereditary component for some types. Patients have paroxysmal hypertension, clammy skin, palpitations, headaches, nausea, and shortness of breath. Diagnosis is by measuring catecholamine products in the blood or urine.

169. C: Meibomian gland. A chalazion usually presents as a painless lump on the upper eyelid. It is due to a blocked meibomian gland. The meibomian glands are also known as tarsal glands and secrete an oily substance. They are located within both the upper and lower eyelid. Chalazion are different from styes, also known as hordeolum, which are usually seen on the lower eyelid and caused by infection. Chalazion generally goes away on its own within months and can be treated with hot compresses.

170. D: 6-9 months. Tuberculosis is caused by acid-fast *Mycobacterium*. Patients may go for periods of time without active infection and have a positive purified protein derivative (PPD) test. Active infection can present with shortness of breath, productive cough, malaise, and night sweats. An upper lobe lung cavitation is characteristic of TB, and diagnosis is by sputum culture. Patients with active infection should avoid spreading disease by covering coughs and avoiding contact with others. For patients with latent infections, Isoniazid (INH) can be given for 6-9 months in order to prevent acute infection.

171. B: Terazosin. This patient has benign prostatic hypertrophy (BPH). The prevalence increases with older age. Patient experience urinary frequency, urgency, dysuria, and nocturia.
Terazosin is an alpha-blocker, which means that it blocks the action of adrenaline and relaxes smooth muscle leading to decreased blockage. Dizziness can be a side effect. Oxybutynin can also treat urinary frequency, but is usually used in urge incontinence.

172. C: Atrial flutter. Atrial flutter is similar to atrial fibrillation in that they are both rapid atrial rhythms and have similar symptoms, but atrial flutter is regular instead of irregular. ECG shows a "sawtooth" pattern. Treatment involves rate control and prevention of thromboembolism. Wolff-Parkinson-White syndrome is a supraventricular tachycardia and "delta waves" are seen on ECG.

173. A: Those who smoke and drink. Around 90% of patients with oral squamous cell carcinoma are smokers. Risk is also increased with heavy alcohol use. Carcinoma of the tongue may be due to syphilis or chronic trauma. Most carcinomas start on the mouth floor or tongue. Detection with screening is important because early lesions may not cause symptoms.

174. A: Lisinopril. This medication is an ACE inhibitor that is often used in the treatment of high blood pressure. Cough is a common side effect. For patients who cannot tolerate this, they are usually switched

to angiotensin receptor blockers instead. Other potential side effects of lisinopril include dizziness, headache, diarrhea, nausea, and hyperkalemia.

175. D: Bacterial meningitis. It involves inflammation of the meninges around the brain or spinal cord. Bacterial meningitis is seen in college age patients due to living in close quarters like dormitories. It is usually caused by meningococci and pneumococci. Vaccine should be considered for students about to leave for college. The classic triad of symptoms is fever, headache, and stiff neck. Brudzinski sign is when hip or knee flexion is induced by neck flexion.

176. B: B12. Dementia is a clinical diagnosis, and distinguishing the type or cause can be difficult. Labs and imaging are ordered to identify treatable causes such as infection, vitamin deficiencies, or toxins. Dementia should also be distinguished from depressive symptoms. Diagnosis of dementia includes one of the following: aphasia, apraxia, agnosia, or executive dysfunction. Other labs that should be ordered in a workup include CBC, CMP, TSH, HIV, RPR, and folate. CT or MRI can also be helpful. Vitamin B12 deficiency can cause cognitive impairment.

177. B: Thiamine. Also known as vitamin B1, thiamine is readily available in a regular diet. However, patients with alcohol dependence are at increased risk for deficiency due to decreased intake, impaired absorption, or increased demand. Thiamine deficiency can lead to polyneuropathy and heart failure. IV glucose can worsen thiamine deficiency, so IV thiamine should always be given first with alcoholic patients.

178. A: Diabetes mellitus. The darkened pigmentation is known as acanthosis nigricans, and it is most often associated with insulin resistance. Acanthosis nigricans can also occur in patients with thyroid disorders, Cushing syndrome, PCOS, or cancer.

179. C: Diarrhea and constipation are uncommon side effects. Anemia is most commonly caused by iron deficiency as a result of blood loss. Blood loss can occur due to occult GI bleeds, menstruation, intravascular hemolysis, or vitamin C deficiency. The cause of anemia should be determined before beginning supplementation. Constipation and diarrhea are common side effects of iron therapy.

180. D: Surgical removal or radiation of pituitary adenoma. Acromegaly describes a condition of excessive growth hormone (GH), usually due to a pituitary adenoma. Patients may present with coarsened facial features, protrusion of the jaw, enlargement of the hands, and thickened body hair. Plasma GH levels will be elevated, and the tumor will be visible by CT or MRI.

181. A: Coarctation of the aorta. This congenital condition is when part of the aorta is narrowed. Symptoms depend on severity and may be present at birth. It can lead to hypertension in the upper extremities, left ventricular hypertrophy, and poor perfusion. Chest x-ray and echocardiography can help the support the diagnosis. Treatment is with balloon angioplasty or surgical correction.

182. B: Pregnancy rate is about 15% in a year of inconsistent condom use. With perfect use, pregnancy rate is about 2% in a year using condoms. Condoms also decrease the risk of sexually transmitted infections. Some condoms are lubricated with a spermicide known as nonoxynol-9. Diaphragms come in different sizes and can be fitted by a health care provider.

183. A: Sialadenitis. This is an infection of a salivary gland, which can occur because of an obstruction or dry mouth. It usually affects the parotid gland and is most commonly caused by *Staphylococcus aureus*. Imaging can confirm diagnosis or show an abscess. It is treated with antibiotics, and patients should use candy to trigger saliva flow. Ludwig angina would involve infection in the tissues below the mouth, and it

is usually bilateral. A peritonsillar abscess would be more apparent when looking into the mouth, rather than seeing external signs.

184. C: Eighth. This is the acoustic or vestibulocochlear cranial nerve. An acoustic neuroma is a tumor of the eighth cranial nerve that leads to hearing loss in the affected ear. The third cranial nerve is the oculomotor cranial nerve. The sixth is the abducens, and the eleventh is the accessory.

185. D: Silicosis. This is a type of pneumoconiosis due to inhalation of silica dust. Quarry workers and sand blasters are at risk. Patients may be asymptomatic at first but eventually develop shortness of breath. Asbestosis is also a type of pneumoconiosis, but chest x-ray would show fibrosis usually in the lower lobes with "honeycombing." Goodpasture syndrome is an autoimmune condition that can cause hemoptysis and is diagnosed by the presence of anti-glomerular basement membrane (GBM) antibodies in the blood.

186. A: Oral steroids. These are usually not used because they do not provide real benefit and may have adverse effects. Steroid injections are sometimes used to relieve pain and increase flexibility. Celecoxib is a COX-2 selective inhibitor, which is a type of NSAID.

187. C: Achalasia. This is a type of motility disorder characterized by lack of peristalsis and incomplete relaxation of the lower esophageal sphincter. On barium x-ray, the esophagus may appear "beaklike" near the lower esophageal sphincter. The exact etiology of achalasia is unknown. Treatment consists of balloon dilation of the sphincter.

188. D: Avascular necrosis. This is a bone infection that can be caused by steroid use, fractures, dislocations, alcohol abuse, tumors, and other diseases. After a trauma, blood supply can become impaired and lead to avascular necrosis (AVN). The "crescent sign" is due to subchondral lucency. The bone collapses and degenerative joint changes occur.

189. B: Decrease the dose. Warfarin is used to prevent thromboembolic events. The medication has potential for many interactions, and the degree of anticoagulation must be monitored closely through blood tests. The international normalized ratio (INR) value for a patient on warfarin should usually be between 2 and 3. If the value is less than 2, then the patient may not be receiving the full benefit of the medication. If the value is greater than 3, then the patient is at increased risk of bleeding.

190. A: Elderly men. Men 75 years and older have the highest rate of death by suicide. Male deaths by suicide outnumber female deaths, although females attempt suicide more. The rate of attempts is high among adolescent females. Firearms are used most often in completed suicides. Factors that increase suicide risk include mental illness, family history of suicide, recent discharge from the hospital, substance use, psychosocial stressors, and previous attempts.

191. A: Bladder carcinoma. Smoking is the most common risk factor. It is more common in men and white people, and incidence increases with age. Bladder cancer is also associated with certain medications and chronic irritation. Patients usually present with hematuria. Polycystic kidney disease is hereditary. The cause is unknown for interstitial cystitis. Kidney stones are not caused by cigarette smoking.

192. C: Histamine release. Urticaria, also known as hives, can be acute or chronic, and has a number of causes. Patients present with erythema and pruritic wheals. It is treated mainly with antihistamines including cetirizine, hydroxyzine, and diphenhydramine.

193. B: Prehypertension. According to the Joint National Committee, blood pressure is considered normal if systolic is below 120 and diastolic is below 80. Prehypertension is a systolic BP between 120-139 or a diastolic BP between 80-89. Stage 1 hypertension is a systolic BP between 140-159 or a diastolic BP between 90-99. Stage 2 hypertension is a systolic BP of 160 or greater or a diastolic BP of 100 or greater. This classification is used for adults 18 years and older. It is based on the average of two or more seated BP readings at two or more office visits.

194. A: Ovarian cancer. CA-125 is a tumor marker that may be elevated in patients with specific types of cancers. It can be used to detect ovarian cancer or to monitor response to treatment, although it is not used as a widespread screening tool because of lack of high sensitivity and specificity. The test can produce false positives and false negatives.

195. D: Nifedipine. Raynaud phenomenon is a vasospastic disorder that affects the fingers or toes. When exposed to cold or stress, skin turns white because of reduced blood flow and then turns blue because of oxygen depletion. Skin eventually turns red as blood flows back in. Patients experience pain and tingling. This phenomenon is often linked to some connective tissue disorders. Calcium channel blockers, such as nifedipine, have been shown to be helpful because they open up blood vessels.

196. B: Oligospermia. Sulfasalazine is a sulfa drug used in the treatment of inflammatory bowel disease. It is thought to be anti-inflammatory and acts as a disease-modifying antirheumatic drug (DMARD). It is also used to treat rheumatoid arthritis. Other potential side effects include GI upset, headache, itching, rash, blood dyscrasia, and hepatotoxicity.

197. A: > 300 mg. Macroalbuminuria is a relatively high rate of urinary excretion of albumin. This means that protein is being leaked that can signify kidney damage or diabetes. It is considered microalbuminuria when the value is between 30 and 300 mg—this is an early sign of progressive cardiovascular and renal disease.

198. D: All of the above. In open reduction and internal fixation (ORIF), reduction refers to how the fracture is realigned, and it can be open or closed. Open reduction means that there is a surgical procedure rather than just closed manipulation or traction. Fixation can be internal or external. Internal fixation involves plates and screws that are put on the bones, compared with external fixation that involves frames and halos.

199. C: Olecranon bursitis. This is an inflammation of the bursa that can occur due to trauma, repetitive stress, or rheumatoid arthritis. Patients present with pain that is worse with increased flexion. It is treated with NSAIDs and activity modification. Sometimes, the bursa will need to be aspirated or surgically excised.

200. D: 40%. An echocardiogram is an ultrasound of the heart. It can be used to evaluate valves, chambers, wall movement, cardiac output, and ejection fraction. The ejection fraction is the amount of blood pumped out of the ventricle with each heartbeat. The normal value is generally between 55% and 70%. Lower ejection fractions manifest clinically as heart failure.

201. A: Increase caffeine intake. Fibrocystic changes are characterized by a benign dense texture and pain of the breasts. Causes include fibrosis, hyperplasia, and cysts. It is more common among women with early menarche or who are nulliparous. It usually presents with bilateral cyclic diffuse pain and engorgement. Studies are mixed regarding the efficacy of dietary modifications used in management, but a possible intervention is to restrict caffeine intake and foods containing methylxanthines. Some women respond to hydrochlorothiazide, and danazol is a synthetic steroid used off-label for treatment.

202. B: Involuntary violent flinging movements of the extremities. Hemiballismus is rare and due to a decrease of subthalamic nucleus activity, which results in decreased suppression of undesired movements. Answer choice A describes bradykinesia, which is usually seen in patients with Parkinson disease. Answer choice C describes chorea of Huntington disease. Answer choice D describes clonus.

203. C: Levonorgestrel. Intrauterine devices (IUDs) are a commonly used method of contraception. It is a T-shaped device and contains levonorgestrel or copper that is released continuously. The IUD renders the uterine environment hostile and prevents fertilization. The IUD lasts for about 5 years. The other answer choices are compounds related to estrogen.

204. C: KUB. Most kidney stones are radiopaque and will show up on x-ray. KUB film stands for kidney, ureter, and bladder. Sometimes a noncontrast spiral CT scan is done or an intravenous pyelogram (IVP), which involves contrast. KUB is less expensive.

205. A: Dacryocystitis. This is due to an obstruction of the nasolacrimal duct. Patients have erythema, edema, and tenderness of the lacrimal sac. Patients may be febrile and have mild conjunctivitis. Treatment is with warm compresses and antibiotics. Surgery may be required to create a fistula for tear flow. Orbital cellulitis would present with edema of the eyelid. Pinguecula occurs on the eye itself, and chalazion usually occurs on the upper eyelid.

206. A: Chloroquine. *Plasmodium ovale* is a species of protozoa that causes malaria. Malaria is caused by four species of *Plasmodium*, and it is spread by mosquitoes. It causes fever and anemia in humans. Possible complications include cerebral disease, pulmonary edema, renal failure, and sepsis. It is especially dangerous in children and pregnant women. Treatment depends on which species is causing the infection and whether antibiotic resistance is present. Chloroquine has been widely used in treatment and prevention.

207. C: Lung crackles. Left-sided heart failure involves pulmonary congestion because fluid backs up in the lungs. Right-sided heart failure causes fluid to accumulate peripherally. Eventually, fluid overload will become generalized with either type of heart failure.

208. A: Croup. This is an acute inflammatory disease involving the upper airway. It is most common in children 3 to 36 months of age. Most cases occur in the fall and winter. Causative agents include parainfluenza, adenovirus, and echovirus. Inspiratory stridor indicates airway obstruction. Bronchiectasis usually has a chronic daily cough with sputum production.

209. B: Younger than 65 years. Valve replacements can be a mechanical prosthetic or biosynthetic. Tissue grafts only have a life expectancy of 10-15 years so they should not be used in younger patients because another operation would be necessary. Mechanical prosthetics require use of warfarin, so pregnant women should have biosynthetic replacement because they cannot take warfarin.

210. C: 25%. Screening for domestic violence in the health care setting should be routine, either by questionnaire or interview. Domestic violence includes intimidation, physical assault, sexual assault, dominance, and abusive behavior. It can result in physical injury, psychological trauma, and even death. About 85% of domestic violence victims are women.

211. A: Diabetes insipidus. This condition is due to deficiency of antidiuretic hormone (ADH), or a nephrogenic cause. Patients present with increased thirst, polyuria, hypernatremia, and dehydration. Diagnosis can be confirmed with 24-hour urine collection, serum labs, and a vasopressin challenge test.

Diabetes insipidus (DI) can present similarly to diabetes mellitus (DM), although elevated glucose would be present with DM.

212. D: Increased PaCO$_2$. Arterial blood gas readings are normally taken from the radial or femoral artery. Parameters that are examined include pH, partial pressure of oxygen, and partial pressure of carbon dioxide. The pH will tell if the patient is acidotic or alkalotic. The lung or kidneys counteract the initial disorder by compensatory mechanism. Respiratory acidosis results from hypoventilation, which causes increased carbon dioxide concentration in the blood and decreased pH. Acidemia is when pH is less than 7.35.

213. C: Physis and metaphysis. Fractures of the growth plate, or physis, in children are described by the Salter-Harris classification system. Salter-Harris I fractures affect the physis only. Salter-Harris II fractures affect the physis and metaphysis. Salter-Harris III fractures affect the physis and epiphysis. Salter-Harris IV fractures affect the physis, metaphysis, and epiphysis. Salter-Harris V fractures are crush injuries.

214. D: Docusate. This is a stool softener that can help the patient avoid straining during bowel movements. This patient likely has hemorrhoids that are caused by dilated veins in the rectum. Patients present with irritation and bleeding. They may become thrombosed or protrude. Treatment can also include warm sitz baths, increased fiber intake, and NSAIDs for pain. In some cases, sclerotherapy or surgery may be required.

215. B: Hypertension. Metoprolol is a beta-blocker and is used to treat angina, stable heart failure, and hypertension. It is contraindicated in patients with sinus bradycardia, second- or third-degree atrioventricular (AV) block, cardiogenic shock, severe peripheral arterial circulatory disorders, and sick sinus syndrome.

216. A: Pleural effusion. This is an accumulation of fluid within the pleural space. There are many causes, including heart failure, cirrhosis, pneumonia, malignancy, pulmonary embolism, tuberculosis, or trauma. Chest x-ray can confirm the diagnosis. Effusions can be classified as transudates or exudates. Pneumothorax is air in the pleural space and would cause hyperresonance to percussion instead of dullness.

217. B: Loss of peripheral vision. Atrophy of the macula is a common cause of worsening vision in elderly patients. The macula is the spot near the center of the retina. Small yellow deposits form under the macula called drusen. Central visual acuity is lost slowly, and central blind spots are called scotomas. Peripheral vision is usually not affected. Macular degeneration is diagnosed by funduscopy and can be treated with laser.

218. B: Teres minor. Injuries of the rotator cuff include strains, tendinitis, and partial or complete tears. The muscles of the rotator cuff are the supraspinatus, infraspinatus, teres minor, and subscapularis. They help stabilize the humerus in the scapula. The rotator cuff cannot be palpated directly, but there are different maneuvers that can be used in the physical exam to test specific muscles for weakness or pain.

219. A: IV nicardipine. This is considered a hypertensive emergency due to a diastolic reading of over 120 and target-organ damage. This can include encephalopathy, preeclampsia, left ventricular failure, MI, renal failure, aortic dissection, and retinopathy. Treatment is with short-acting IV drugs used to progressively lower blood pressure with titration. Nicardipine is a calcium channel blocker and acts as a vasodilator. Other drugs used include nitroprusside, labetalol, and fenoldopam. Onset is more variable with oral drugs.

220. D: Decreased deep tendon reflexes. Myasthenia gravis is an autoimmune neuromuscular disease characterized by muscle fatigability. Antibodies block acetylcholine receptors, so it is treated with acetylcholinesterase inhibitors. Patients have weakness of the eye muscles and of the limbs. More severe disease can affect the respiratory muscles. Deep tendon reflexes are usually preserved.

221. B: Call surgery. This patient is presenting with appendicitis, which is most common in teenagers and patients in their 20s. Patients usually have periumbilical pain at first, which then shifts to the right lower quadrant. McBurney point is located at one-third of the distance from the anterior superior iliac spine to the umbilicus. Gangrene and perforation can occur if left untreated, so it is considered an emergency.

222. C: Polycystic kidney disease. This is a progressive genetic condition that may be asymptomatic at first but patients may present with symptoms while in their 20s. It can be autosomal dominant or recessive. Patients present with flank pain, hematuria, and hypertension. It is diagnosed by CT or ultrasound. It may progress to renal failure and require dialysis or transplantation. Patients can have extrarenal manifestations such as hepatic cysts, valvular heart disorders, or cerebral aneurysms.

223. D: Triamcinolone. Lichen simplex chronicus is characterized by darkened, leathery-appearing skin due to repeated scratching. It occurs frequently in patients with anxiety disorders. Dry, scaling plaques are usually seen on the legs, arms, neck, and trunk. It may appear similarly to tinea, lichen planus, and psoriasis. Treatment is with topical steroids.

224. C: Hodgkin lymphoma. Also known as Hodgkin disease, this is a malignant proliferation of cells of the lymphoreticular system. Patients may present with lymphadenopathy, fever, weight loss, splenomegaly, or hepatomegaly. It is diagnosed through biopsy and treated with chemotherapy and radiation. Reed-Sternberg cells are large and binucleated—they are abnormal cells that result from clonal transformation of B lymphocytes.

225. D: Selective serotonin reuptake inhibitor. Also know as an SSRI, fluvoxamine works by inhibiting the reuptake of serotonin into the presynaptic cell so that more serotonin is available in the synaptic cleft to bind to the postsynaptic receptor. Serotonin is a neurotransmitter found in the brain that is thought to help regulate mood. SSRIs are used in the treatment of depression and anxiety. Other SSRIs include citalopram, fluoxetine, paroxetine, and sertraline.

226. B: Type I diabetes mellitus. This usually develops in children and adolescents and is considered insulin-dependent, whereas type II diabetes develops more often in adults who may or may not need insulin replacement. In type I diabetes, insulin production is absent because of autoimmune destruction of pancreatic B cells. Patients may present in diabetic ketoacidosis, which is an acute complication characterized by hyperglycemia.

227. A: Polymorphic ventricular tachycardia associated with long QT syndrome. In torsades de pointes, the ventricular rate can range from 150-250 beats per minute. It appears on ECG as irregular twisting of the QRS complex around the baseline. Prolonged QT interval, which is inherited or caused by medications, predisposes individuals to arrhythmias that can trigger torsades. Torsades can terminate spontaneously or may degenerate into ventricular fibrillation, which can lead to sudden death without intervention.

228. C: *Streptococcus pneumoniae*. Pneumonia is an inflammation of the lungs that can be caused by bacteria, viruses, fungi, or parasites. Many pathogens present similarly in patients, and it is often difficult or unnecessary to determine the specific causative agent. Chest x-ray will usually show an infiltrate. *Streptococcus pneumoniae, Haemophilus influenzae, Mycoplasma pneumoniae,* and *Chlamydia pneumoniae*

are the most common bacterial causes. Adenovirus is a common infection but usually does not cause pneumonia. *Histoplasma capsulatum* is a fungus that causes infection more commonly in patients with weakened immune systems. RSV infection usually occurs in children.

229. A: 32-year-old African-American woman. Sarcoidosis is characterized by noncaseating granulomas found in organs and tissues. The etiology is unknown. Diagnosis is usually first suspected because of lung involvement. It primarily affects people 20-40 years of age, and prevalence is greatest in northern Europeans and in people of African descent in the United States. It is slightly more prevalent in women.

230. B: Optic chiasm. The pituitary gland is located in the sella turcica, which is a fossa of the sphenoid bone. A pituitary adenoma may present with visual field defects due to compression of the optic nerve. The optic chiasm is the area where the optic nerves partially cross, making an "x." Pressure on the optic chiasm can cause bitemporal hemianopia, which is a bilateral temporal visual field defect.

231. D: Albuterol. Citalopram is an SSRI used for depression and anxiety. GI upset is a common side effect, in the form of nausea, vomiting, or diarrhea. Gastrointestinal upset is common when metformin is first prescribed for treatment of diabetes. Naproxen is an NSAID and can cause heartburn and ulcers. Albuterol is used in the treatment of asthma and does not typically have GI side effects.

232. B: Homan sign. This patient likely has a deep venous thrombosis (DVT), which is a blood clot usually occurring in a deep vein of the calf or thigh. Risk factors include recent surgery, immobilization, smoking, heart failure, trauma, obesity, malignancy, contraceptive use, and pregnancy. DVTs cause pain and swelling and can lead to pulmonary embolism. They are treated with anticoagulants. Homan sign is when ankle dorsiflexion elicits calf pain when the knee is extended. The sign is neither sensitive nor specific, but it can occur with distal leg DVTs.

233. D: 40. In 2011, the ACOG revised its screening guideline to recommend that mammography should be offered annually to women starting at age 40. The previous recommendation was that mammograms be done every 1 or 2 years starting at age 40 and then annually beginning at age 50. This new guideline differs from the guideline of the United States Preventive Services Task Force, which recommends that biennial mammography be done from ages 50-74.

234. A: Prostaglandins. The cause of primary pulmonary hypertension (PPH) is unknown. Pulmonary vessels become constricted and fibrosed, leading to right ventricular failure. Patients present with fatigue and exertional dyspnea. Tests may be obtained to rule out secondary causes. PPH is diagnosed by measuring pulmonary artery pressure. Prostaglandins are used as treatment because they dilate vessels. Some patients may require transplantation.

235. B: Detrusor. This muscle contracts when urinating. Involuntary bladder contractions are caused by overactivity of the detrusor muscle. This is a type of urge incontinence commonly seen in elderly women. Treatment can include bladder training, Kegel exercises, and relaxation techniques. Oxybutynin can suppress urgency symptoms.

236. C: Transient ischemic attack. A TIA is similar to a stroke but the symptoms last less than an hour. TIAs do increase risk of stroke. This patient likely experienced amaurosis fugax, which is transient monocular blindness caused by ischemia of the ophthalmic artery. When TIAs occur, it is important to test for hemorrhage, carotid stenosis, and arrhythmias. Antiplatelet drugs are given to prevent strokes. Central retinal artery occlusions also cause unilateral blindness, but vision does not usually improve. Optic neuritis presents with pain.

237. A: Radial deviation of the fingers. Rheumatoid arthritis is a chronic systemic inflammatory disease that mainly affects the joints. Patients with rheumatoid arthritis have ulnar deviation of the fingers. Boutonniere deformity is when the proximal interphalangeal joints are flexed and the distal interphalangeal joints are hyperextended. Keratoconjunctivitis sicca is eye dryness. Anti-citrullinated peptide antibodies have a high specificity and sensitivity for RA.

238. B: Achilles tendon rupture. This tendon connects the calf muscles to the heel, so that the foot can be plantar flexed. Athletes or patients who have been inactive for a period may be more prone to rupture. Quinolone antibiotics have also been associated with an increased risk of rupture. A positive Thompson test means that the foot does not plantar flex when you squeeze the calf muscle while the patient is lying prone with their feet hanging off the table.

239. B: Fenofibrate. This is a fibrate medication that works well to reduce triglycerides. Although it can potentiate muscle toxicity when used in conjunction with a statin, this combination can provide a significant therapeutic advantage for refractory hyperlipidemia. Statins work well to reduce LDL and reduce cardiovascular mortality. They also provide small increases in HDL and modest decreases in triglycerides. It would not be much more helpful to add another statin to the patient's regimen, such as rosuvastatin. Bile acid sequestrants, such as colestipol and cholestyramine, may actually increase triglyceride levels.

240. A: NSAIDs. This patient likely has De Quervain thyroiditis, also known as subacute thyroiditis. It is an acute inflammation of the thyroid likely due to a viral infection. Patients present with fever and thyroid tenderness. Thyroid function tests (TFTs) may initially show hyperthyroidism. It can be distinguished from Graves disease through the radioactive iodine uptake test, since Graves will result in increased uptake. De Quervain thyroiditis resolves within months. It is treated with high doses of NSAIDs or steroids.

241. D: All of the above. The coronary arteries supply oxygen-rich blood to the myocardium. The arteries originate from the aorta, stemming off just after the aorta exits the left ventricle. There is some variation from person to person as to the exact number or placement of coronary arteries.

242. C: Determining whether Vitamin B12 is being absorbed normally. The test is done in several different stages, where patients are given radioactive and nonradioactive B12 orally and by injection and then in combination with other substances. Urine is collected to measure if Vitamin B12 is normally absorbed. Low B12 can occur from lack of intrinsic factor due to pernicious anemia, malabsorption, bacterial overgrowth, or pancreatic insufficiency. Answer choice A describes the Coombs test. Answer choice B is related to the total iron binding capacity, and answer choice D describes hemoglobin electrophoresis.

243. A: Hepatitis A. This is spread by the fecal-oral route and can be transmitted through contaminated food or water. Infections are self-limited and confer immunity to reinfection. There is no specific treatment. IgM antibodies are present with acute infection, and IgG antibodies persist afterwards, signifying immunity. IgG antibodies are also found in the blood after vaccination. HBV is usually transmitted through blood or sex, and HCV is commonly transmitted through blood. Hepatitis D is less common and co-occurs with HBV.

244. C: Previous cesarean sections. Placenta previa is an obstetric complication in which the placenta is implanted in the lower part of the uterus near the internal os. It usually happens during the second or third trimester and can lead to bright red vaginal bleeding. The exact cause is unknown although several risk factors have been identified. These include previous uterine damage (multiple pregnancies,

abnormalities, surgeries, cesarean deliveries), smoking during pregnancy, increased maternal age, and twin pregnancy.

245. C: Cognitive and memory dysfunction. Electroconvulsive therapy (ECT) is a psychiatric treatment in which seizures are induced in anesthetized patients. It is used for treatment of severe depression that has not responded to other modalities. The exact mechanism for how it works remains unknown. Proper informed consent should be obtained prior to the procedure.

246. A: Moxifloxacin. Conjunctivitis, also known as pink eye, is inflammation that can be caused by bacteria, viruses, or allergies. This patient likely has bacterial conjunctivitis due to the presence of purulent eye discharge. It is commonly caused by staphylococci or streptococci, and is highly contagious. Viral conjunctivitis usually presents with watery discharge and lymphadenopathy. Steroids may be helpful, and povidone-iodine (*Betadine*) is sometimes used off-label in treatment. Allergic conjunctivitis would be bilateral and accompanied by other allergy symptoms such as itchy eyes, congestion, and sneezing. It can be alleviated with antihistamines such as olopatadine.

247. B: 2 months. The DTaP vaccine combines protection against diphtheria, tetanus, and pertussis. The first dose is given at the age of 2 months, with additional doses at 4 months, 6 months, 15-18 months, and 4-6 years.

248. C: Inadequate cellular oxygen supply. The causes of shock may differ (decreased blood volume, decreased cardiac output, vasodilation) but the pathophysiology is the same. Patients with low blood pressure are not necessarily in shock, although low blood pressure can be a sign of shock. Shock is hypoperfusion of vital tissues that causes inadequate oxygen supply so that cells shift to anaerobic metabolism, leading to accumulation of lactic acid and cellular dysfunction. The body makes attempts to compensate, including vasoconstriction and increased retention of water and sodium. Patients can present with altered mental status, tachycardia, tachypnea, cyanosis, diaphoresis, and weak pulses. Persistent shock leads to irreversible damage and cell death.

249. A: 15-20 weeks. Maternal serum screening can identify women at increased risk of having a child with a neural tube defect, Down syndrome, or trisomy 18. Elevated levels of maternal alpha-fetoprotein suggest spina bifida or anencephaly. The "triple screen" can detect risk of Down syndrome by testing alpha-fetoprotein, beta-human chorionic gonadotropin, and estriol. Some labs include inhibin A for a "quad screen."

250. D: Foreign body aspiration. Obstruction with a foreign body will cause marked resistance when doing mouth-to-mouth or bag ventilation. If the object is not able to be removed in the oropharynx, then the Heimlich maneuver or chest compressions will need to be done.

251. C: Mycophenolate. This medication is an immunosuppressant used to prevent organ transplant rejection. Certain medications can cause subtle injury to the kidneys or overt renal failure. The kidney's role in filtration exposes cells to significant concentrations of drugs, which can lead to changes in function and structure. Damage can be reversible or chronic. Gentamicin and amphotericin B can cause tubular toxicity, and penicillin can cause interstitial inflammation.

252. D: Mitral regurgitation. This is when the mitral valve between the left atrium and left ventricle is incompetent, so that blood flows backwards during systole. Rheumatic fever is a common cause for this condition. Aortic stenosis produces a crescendo-decrescendo ejection murmur best heard at the left upper sternal border. Aortic regurgitation is when blood is flowing in the wrong direction from the aorta

back into the left ventricle—it would cause a diastolic murmur. Mitral stenosis is a narrowing of the valve between the left atrium and left ventricle, and the rumbling murmur would also occur during diastole.

253. A: 5%. Patients with pancreatic cancer present with abdominal pain, loss of appetite, weight loss, and jaundice. They have a poor prognosis because disease is often advanced when they are diagnosed. The majority of patients are surgically unresectable. Symptomatic treatment is important. Depending on the stage of cancer, 5-year survival rate is roughly between 1% and 15%. If the cancer is localized and able to be removed surgically, 5-year survival rate can approach 25%.

254. C: Cranial nerve VIII – vestibulocochlear. Cranial nerve I is the olfactory nerve, and cranial nerve IV is the trochlear nerve. The optic nerve is cranial nerve II, and the trigeminal nerve is cranial nerve V.

255. B: 100-125 mg/dL. A patient is considered to have impaired fasting glucose if the lab value is between 100 and 125 mg/dL. This is also known as pre-diabetes. Less than 100 mg/dL is considered normal. Diabetes can be diagnosed if fasting plasma glucose is 126 mg/dL or greater, if oral glucose tolerance test is 200 mg/dL or greater, or if hemoglobin $A_{1c}$ is 6.5% or greater.

256. D: Compartment syndrome. This occurs usually after an injury when bleeding or swelling of the tissues increases pressure within a compartment of the body. The fascia layers do not stretch, so blood flow is compromised, which can cause ischemia and lead to further edema. Compartment syndrome presents similarly to peripheral arterial disease, in that there can be paresthesia, pallor, and pulselessness. However, with compartment syndrome the pain is usually out of proportion to what is expected. It is an emergency and requires fasciotomy to relieve the pressure.

257. A: Ribavirin. Human immunodeficiency virus (HIV) destroys CD4 lymphocytes and impairs cell-mediated immunity, thus making patients more vulnerable to other infections. Treatment is often a combination of several drugs in order to suppress virus replication. With successful therapy, HIV RNA becomes undetectable. Ribavirin is an antiviral drug, but it is used to treat hepatitis C.

258. B: 8%. Asthma is a condition in which the airway becomes inflamed, leading to bronchoconstriction. The prevalence has increased continuously since the 1970s, with possible causes being changes in lifestyle and environment. Asthma is the most common chronic condition among children.

259. A: Squat. Aortic stenosis is narrowing of the aortic valve, which will produce a crescendo-decrescendo murmur with systole. It is best heard at the left upper sternal border when the patient is leaning forward. The murmur of aortic stenosis typically increases with maneuvers that increase left ventricular volume, such as leg raising and squatting. The murmur decreases with the Valsalva maneuver, which decreases left ventricular volume, and the murmur also decreases with isometric handgrip due to increased afterload.

260. D: Omeprazole. This patient likely has uncomplicated gastroesophageal reflux disease (GERD), which is a common condition due to lower esophageal sphincter incompetence. Patients present with burning pain due to reflux of gastric contents. Fatty foods, caffeine, alcohol, and weight gain can make GERD worse. Omeprazole is a proton pump inhibitor that reduces gastric acid secretion. Patients should also be advised to elevate the head of their bed and avoid eating close to bedtime.

261. C: Preterm labor. Amniocentesis is an obstetrical procedure in which fluid is withdrawn from the amniotic sac for a variety of tests. It is performed with a needle under ultrasound guidance. Amniocentesis can cause bleeding, infection, preterm labor, or fetal injury/loss.

262. B: Side effect from medication. Since this patient has schizoaffective disorder, he is likely taking an antipsychotic medication. One of the potential side effects with this class of medications is tardive dyskinesia. This manifests as involuntary abnormal movements of the lips, jaw, tongue, neck, hips, arms, or legs. It can persist even after the medication is stopped. The rating instrument called the Abnormal Involuntary Movement Scale (AIMS) can be used for evaluation.

263. A: Lidocaine. Insects in the ear are most irritating while they are still alive. Filling the ear canal with viscous lidocaine will kill the insect, which can then be removed with forceps.

264. C: Polymyositis. This is a chronic inflammation of the muscles. The exact cause is unknown, although there is an autoimmune component. It occurs more often in females. Patients present with pain, symmetric weakness, and loss of muscle mass. It can be complicated by malignancy. Polymyositis is treated with steroids. It may present similarly to other autoimmune conditions. It is related to dermatomyositis, although this condition includes skin manifestations. Guillain-Barré syndrome also presents with symmetrical weakness, although this condition affects the nervous system.

265. B: Varenicline. Patients are encouraged to set a "quit date" and then start taking this medication 1 week prior, or patients can start taking varenicline and then quit smoking between day 8 and 35 of treatment. The dose is titrated up to 1 mg twice daily, and treatment continues for 12 weeks. The medication is an alpha4-beta2 nicotinic acetylcholine receptor partial agonist. Disulfiram and acamprosate are used for alcohol dependence, and buprenorphine is used for opioid dependence.

266. D: Gastrus. The stomach is divided into four regions. The cardia surrounds the opening of the esophagus into the stomach. The fundus forms the upper curvature and is above the level of the cardial orifice. The body is the main largest region. The pylorus is the lower section where contents are about to be emptied into the small intestine.

267. A: Hernia. This is a protrusion of the abdominal contents through a weakness in the abdominal wall. This patient has an umbilical hernia. They are usually asymptomatic and can be treated with elective surgery. Sometimes umbilical hernias can be painful because of strangulation (compromise of the blood supply to its hernial contents).

268. C: Oxygen. Bronchiolitis is an inflammation of the bronchioles, usually caused by viruses such as RSV. The virus causes epithelial necrosis and leads to obstruction and air trapping. It mostly affects children younger than 18 months. Patients can have coughing, wheezing, dyspnea, poor feeding, retractions, and crackles. Chest x-ray would show hyperinflation. Treatment is supportive and can include oxygen and hydration. There is some evidence that epinephrine may provide relief as a bronchodilator. Antibiotics are not indicated unless there is an overlying bacterial infection suggested.

269. B: Hoarseness. This is due to damage of the recurrent laryngeal nerve, which ascends between the trachea and esophagus and passes near the thyroid gland to enter the larynx.
Removal of the thyroid gland can result in hypothyroidism depending on the extent of the surgery. It can also cause hypoparathyroidism because the parathyroid glands are close by and may be damaged.

270. D: 1-2. Urine pregnancy tests check for the presence of human chorionic gonadotropin, which is produced in a growing placenta after implantation. The time it takes for a fertilized egg to implant in the uterus varies among women. It usually takes 6-12 days. Urine pregnancy tests are best done in the morning so that the urine is most concentrated. Tests can be falsely negative if done too early after conception. Blood pregnancy tests can usually show results earlier than urine pregnancy tests.

271. C: Order a sleep study. This patient likely has obstructive sleep apnea (OSA) that can be diagnosed with polysomnography. This is an interruption of breathing while sleeping. Apnea causes a suffocating sensation that does not usually wake the patient, but is enough to let breathing begin again. Risk factors include obesity and family history. OSA is associated with hypertension and diabetes. Patients with OSA often report snoring, gasping/choking sensation during the night, and daytime fatigue. Treatment is with positive airway pressure. Use of the sedative zolpidem can worsen untreated sleep apnea. Modafinil acts as a stimulant and can improve daytime fatigue, but underlying OSA should be treated first.

272. D: Borderline. This personality disorder is in Cluster B on Axis II, as described in the *Diagnostic and Statistical Manual of Mental Disorders, Fourth Edition*. Borderline personality disorder (BPD) is characterized by a pervasive pattern of instability and impulsiveness. Patients make efforts to avoid abandonment, have unstable relationships with extremes between idealization and devaluation, feel empty, and make recurrent suicidal gestures.

273. C: Have her undergo Holter monitoring. Holter monitoring is continuous monitoring and recording of the ECG. It is useful for evaluation of intermittent arrhythmias that may not show up on a one-time physical exam. Patients wear the device for 24 hours and are also asked to record their symptoms so that they can be correlated with the data.

274. D: Carisoprodol. Risedronate and zoledronic acid are bisphosphonates that work by inhibiting bone resorption. Raloxifene is a selective estrogen receptor modulator that decreases bone turnover and increases bone mineral density. Carisoprodol is a muscle relaxant.

275. A: Pia mater, subarachnoid space, arachnoid mater, dura mater. The spinal canal lies within a bony canal. The anterior wall is formed by the vertebrae, discs, and ligaments. The vertebral arches and ligaments cover the other sides. Within the vertebral canal, the spinal cord is surrounded by the meninges. The subarachnoid space contains cerebrospinal fluid. Outside of the dura mater is the epidural space containing tissues, fat, and vessels.

276. D: Instruct patient to overcook food so that folate is preserved. Deficiency of folic acid can be due to inadequate dietary intake, malabsorption, decreased metabolism, or drug interactions. Folate is found in citrus fruits, meats, and green leafy vegetables. Prolonged cooking actually destroys folate. Folate deficiency can cause megaloblastic anemia. Folate is important for DNA synthesis, and deficiency results in decreased RBC life.

277. B: Walls off inflammation. The greater omentum is a large double-layered membrane that attaches to the stomach and duodenum. It drapes over the intestines and colon and lies freely suspended. It contains fat and vessels. It tends to "migrate" to inflamed areas and wrap itself around, adhering to diseased areas of the bowel.

278. C: Two pulmonary arteries. The root of each lung consists of structures that attach to the mediastinum. It is surrounded by pleura and this region is known as the hilum. One pulmonary artery, two pulmonary veins, a main bronchus, bronchial vessels, nerves, and lymphatics are within each lung root and located in the hilum.

279. B: Herpes keratitis. This is the leading cause of infectious corneal blindness in the United States. It is caused by HSV and transmitted through bodily fluids. The virus replicates in the corneal epithelium and breaks it down. Herpes keratitis produces hallmark dendritic ulcers.

280. B: Breast cancer. This patient has what is called "peau d'orange" that means that tumor growth and lymphatic obstruction can pull on the connective tissue in the breast to give the dimpled appearance of an orange peel. Breast cancer is one of the most common malignancies in women. This patient will need to have a biopsy and staging. There is also concern for metastases because it is unknown how long the cancer has been present.

281. D: Nephrotic syndrome. This is a condition in which the kidneys leak protein into the urine because of increased permeability of the glomerular capillary wall. It may be the result of kidney disease or from another systemic condition that affects the kidneys. It is diagnosed by 24-hour urine collection when excretion of protein is greater than 3.5 g. It is treated with fluid restriction, diet, diuretics, and ACE inhibitors.

282. C: Thoracentesis. This is when the chest wall is punctured for aspiration of pleural fluid. Pleural effusion is an accumulation of fluid within the pleural space due to many causes. Chest x-ray can confirm the diagnosis. Thoracentesis can determine the etiology of the pleural effusion or relieve dyspnea. A paracentesis is when the peritoneal cavity is punctured, usually for relief of ascites. Physiotherapy consists of external maneuvers to clear airway secretions as in cystic fibrosis.

283. A: Obesity. Endometrial cancer primarily affects postmenopausal women and typically presents with vaginal bleeding. Risk factors include obesity, diabetes, hypertension, unopposed estrogen (associated with nulliparity, early menarche, late menopause, anovulation, and estrogen therapy), family history of breast or ovarian cancer, and prior pelvic radiation therapy. Endometrial cancer is diagnosed by biopsy.

284. C: Chest wall disease. Pulmonary function tests (PFTs) are used to evaluate functional change in a patient with known or suspected lung disease. PFTs provide information on lung volumes, flow rates, and gas transfer. An obstructive pattern means that there is a decrease in rates of expiratory airflow and air trapping. This is seen with asthma, chronic bronchitis, and emphysema. A restrictive pattern is seen in neuromuscular and chest wall diseases, which means that there is a reduction in lung volume and normal expiratory airflow.

285. D: Stomach cancer. Carcinoma of the stomach is a common gastrointestinal malignancy. *Helicobacter pylori* plays a significant role in the cause of stomach cancer. Gastric polyps can also be precursors of cancer. Symptoms can include epigastric pain, early satiety, bleeding, and obstruction. Surgical resection is possible if diagnosed early, but many patients present with advanced disease.

286. B: Perineal body. This is a connective tissue structure where muscles of the pelvic floor and perineum attach, including the levator ani, deep transverse perineal, superficial transverse perineal, external anal sphincter, sphincter urethrovaginalis, and bulbospongiosus muscles. The perineal body may be stretched and torn during childbirth, so an obstetrician may preemptively make an incision in the perineal body known as a midline episiotomy.

287. A: Banding of varices. An upper endoscopy (esophagogastroduodenoscopy or EGD) is a procedure in which a tube with a camera is inserted into the patient's mouth, in order to examine the esophagus, stomach, duodenum, and proximal jejunum. The mucosa can be directly visualized. Abnormal areas can be biopsied, and bleeding can be cauterized. Upper endoscopy can be used for banding of varices, dilation of strictures, removal of a foreign body, and surveillance of ulcers.

288. C: Leukotriene receptor antagonist. This medication is used for prophylaxis and long-term treatment of asthma and for prevention of exercise-induced bronchoconstriction. It is not used as primary treatment of acute attacks. It can also relieve symptoms of seasonal allergies.

289. B: Consolidation. Tactile fremitus is the palpable vibration of the chest wall that results from vocalization. The patient is asked to recite numbers or words while the examiner systematically palpates the chest with the ulnar aspects of the hands. Tactile fremitus is increased with the presence of fluids or a solid mass within the lungs, usually from consolidation, secretions, or tumors. Tactile fremitus is decreased because of excess air in the lungs or bronchial obstruction.

290. D: Acute lymphoblastic leukemia. ALL is a malignant proliferation of lymphoid stem cells that occurs mainly in children. The exact cause is unknown. Patients present with fever, fatigue, weight loss, bone pain, and bleeding. Chemotherapy has a high success rate. Chronic lymphocytic leukemia (CLL), acute myelogenous leukemia (AML), and chronic myelogenous leukemia (CML) usually occur in adults older than 50 years.

291. C: Stimulants. This patient likely has attention deficit hyperactivity disorder (ADHD), which is a characterized by inattention, hyperactivity, or both. Patients have difficulty following instructions, are distractible, make careless mistakes, have a hard time organizing, and are restless. In addition to behavioral interventions and school support, stimulant medications have been shown to be helpful in reducing symptoms.

292. A: L3 and L4. The needle can be inserted between L3 and L4 or between L4 and L5—these sites are below the termination of the spinal cord. The patient is placed in the lateral or prone position. The needle is passed in between the spinous processes into the epidural space, and further advancement punctures the dura and arachnoid matter. The needle enters the subarachnoid space and usually pushes away the spinal nerve roots without problems. Then cerebrospinal fluid can be aspirated for analysis.

293. B: Papillary. This accounts for 70% to 80% of thyroid cancers. It is usually seen in women 30-60 years of age. Most thyroid cancers present as asymptomatic nodules, and diagnosis is by fine-needle aspiration biopsy. Treatment is by surgical removal. Follicular and anaplastic carcinoma are more common among elderly patients. Medullary carcinoma is often familial.

294. D: Kyphosis. This is an abnormal curvature of the vertebral column in the thoracic region. It can be caused by osteoporosis in elderly patients, producing a "dowager's hump." Scoliosis is an abnormal lateral curvature along with a rotational element. It may be present at birth or be a manifestation of a nerve condition, tumor, or disc protrusion. Lordosis is an abnormal curvature in the lumbar region, which is also called a swayback deformity.

295. A: Fluconazole. Cryptococcosis is a fungal infection usually seen in AIDS patients and other immunocompromised patients. Pulmonary infection may present with fever, cough, and shortness of breath. The infection can disseminate to the skin, meninges, joints, and internal organs. It is diagnosed by culture. The antifungal medications fluconazole or amphotericin B are used in treatment depending on the severity and spread of disease. Patients who are immunocompetent may not require treatment for localized pulmonary infection.

296. A: Glaucoma. Tonometry is used to measure intraocular pressure. Different types of tonometers are used by eye care professionals. Glaucoma is a disease of the optic nerve related to abnormal drainage of aqueous humor, which can cause increased ocular pressure. This results in decreased vision in the peripheral fields and potential blindness.

297. B: No other intervention needed at this time. This patient likely has a Mallory-Weiss tear, which is a superficial tear at the gastroesophageal junction caused by vomiting. The bleeding will usually stop on its own and will not require intervention.

298. D: 0.6–1.2 mEq/L. Lithium is used in the treatment of bipolar disorder. Serum lithium levels must be monitored to avoid toxicity. The lab should be drawn 8-12 hours after the patient's last dose. Thyroid and renal function should also be monitored.

299. B: Trichomoniasis. This is a sexually transmitted infection with the protozoan *Trichomonas vaginalis*. Men are usually asymptomatic, or they may have urethritis resulting in discharge or dysuria. The organism is harder to detect in men than women. It is treated with metronidazole. Giardiasis is also caused by a flagellated protozoan, but this organism causes infection of the gastrointestinal tract.

300. A: Cirrhosis. This is a liver disorder that can be confirmed histologically. It is characterized by widespread fibrosis due to cell damage. Causes include long-term alcohol abuse, chronic hepatitis B or C infection, biliary obstruction, and malnutrition. Increased pressure in the portal vein leads to splenomegaly and varicose veins. Progressive liver failure leads to fluid retention producing ascites. The inability to break down blood products manifests as jaundice. Patients are more at risk of bleeding because of decreased production of clotting proteins.